TOXIC DISRUPTIONS

This book provides a unique ethnographic account of women living with polycystic ovary syndrome (PCOS) in India. It examines how contaminated environments and political–economic changes render urban middle-class women in India vulnerable to PCOS, a condition which has the potential to disrupt conventional, normative feminine biographies of marriage and childbearing.

The volume revolves around two main themes: how toxic landscapes, the endocrine disrupting chemicals suffusing them, and the political–economic environments related to them are linked to endocrine disorders such as PCOS; and how the biosocial disruptions caused by PCOS are both affecting women and reflective of changes in contemporary urban India. The author draws on anthropological fieldwork to investigate these connections through a fresh approach, combining a political ecological framework with perspectives from the anthropology of toxic exposures and health–environment systems.

The first of its kind, this volume will be indispensable to students and researchers of anthropology, particularly medical anthropology, medical sociology, human geography, science and technology studies, medical humanities, health–environment systems, endocrine disorders, public health, and South Asian studies.

Gauri Pathak is a medical anthropologist and associate professor at the Department of Global Studies, Aarhus University, Denmark. Her research focuses on the interactions between the body and its environment, consumption practices, and processes of globalization in South Asia, especially urban India. A former Homi Bhabha fellow, she is a founding member of the Plastic Lives social science consortium, and her current project, supported by a Carlsberg Young Researcher Fellowship, revolves around ethnographic investigations of human–plastic entanglements and the resulting toxic exposures. Besides her work on plastics and the lived experiences of polycystic ovary syndrome, she has also investigated beauty work and body projects in urban India.

TOXIC DISRUPTIONS

Polycystic Ovary Syndrome in Urban India

Gauri Pathak

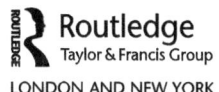

Routledge
Taylor & Francis Group
LONDON AND NEW YORK

First published 2023
by Informa Law from Routledge
4 Park Square, Milton Park, Abingdon, Oxon OX14 4RN

and by Informa Law from Routledge
605 Third Avenue, New York, NY 10158

Informa Law from Routledge is an imprint of the Taylor & Francis Group, an informa business

British Library Cataloguing-in-Publication Data
A catalogue record for this book is available from the British Library

Library of Congress Cataloging-in-Publication Data
Names: Pathak, Gauri, author.
Title: Toxic disruptions : polycystic ovary syndrome in urban India / Gauri Pathak.
Description: First edition. | Abingdon, Oxon ; New York : Informa Law from Routledge, an imprint of the Taylor & Francis Group, 2023. | Includes bibliographical references and index.
Identifiers: LCCN 2022041301 (print) | LCCN 2022041302 (ebook) | ISBN 9780367774462 (hbk) | ISBN 9780367774479 (pbk) | ISBN 9781003171423 (ebk)
Subjects: LCSH: Polycystic ovary syndrome--India. | Endocrine disrupting chemicals--Health aspects--India.
Classification: LCC RG480.S7 P385 2023 (print) | LCC RG480.S7 (ebook) | DDC 618.1/100954--dc23/eng/20220929
LC record available at https://lccn.loc.gov/2022041301
LC ebook record available at https://lccn.loc.gov/2022041302

ISBN: 978-0-367-77446-2 (hbk)
ISBN: 978-0-367-77447-9 (pbk)
ISBN: 978-1-003-17142-3 (ebk)

DOI: 10.4324/9781003171423

Typeset in Sabon
by SPi Technologies India Pvt Ltd (Straive)

CONTENTS

ACKNOWLEDGMENTS

This book would never have been written without support from a host of people. Above all, I am deeply grateful to all my interlocutors for allowing me into their lives and sharing so generously of themselves. Without them, there would be nothing to write about.

I would also like to thank the members of my PhD committee for their support and advice throughout the evolution of the dissertation that was the first incarnation of this book. Mark and Mimi Nichter have continued to be advisors far beyond the PhD. I'm not sure what karmic twist led me to them, but I am forever indebted. Despite multiple demands on their time, they somehow always manage to make time to engage in hours-long discussions, provide comprehensive inputs, and offer unwavering support. They have challenged me to grow both intellectually and as a person, and they have been true gurus, in every sense of the word. Brian Silverstein could be relied upon to have an interesting point of view, and he provided thoughtful advice and a wonderful sense of humor. Susan Shaw was always ready with constructive feedback and important insights.

Several others have critically engaged with the ideas presented in the pages that follow. Marcia Inhorn provided invaluable inputs and advice. Isha Dubey read and commented on early versions of the manuscript. Conversations with Atreyee Sen, Emery Eaves, Manuela Ciotti, Priscilla Magrath, Shashank Dengle, and Kim Kelly helped me refine my arguments. The ideas contained in this book have been presented at various seminars, conferences, and workshops at the University of Arizona, Aarhus University, Yale University, the University of Oslo, Copenhagen University, and the Indian Institute of Technology, Hyderabad. This book is much better for the discussions that ensued and critical engagements from participants. I am also grateful for feedback from the anonymous peer reviewers who read and commented on not just the manuscript but also the book proposal.

In Mumbai, a number of people, both family and friends, formed my support system as I conducted the fieldwork. My thanks to Smita Rao, Urmi Palan, Sapna Punjabi, Mihir Patkar, Gayatri Sarang, Ashish Rao, Raju Kane, Tanvir Gill, Smruthy Nair, Belinda Vaz, Utsav Mamoria, Juilee Katkar, Sonalia Fernandes-Soans, Rahat Shaikh, Sunil Naik, and Savita Naik, who good-naturedly allowed me to pester them for contacts and tap them as resources. Very special thanks to Narendra Palan, without whom the comprehensive interviews with medical practitioners would never have been possible.

Funding from the School of Anthropology at the University of Arizona and later the School of Culture and Society at Aarhus University enabled the fieldwork. I am also grateful to the research program at the Department of Global Studies, Aarhus University, for support with publication.

Being a part of the Department of Global Studies at Aarhus University has provided me with the stimulating academic environment that proved crucial during the final stages of writing this book. In particular, I am grateful for the intellectual and personal friendship of Anemone Platz, Annette Skovsted Hansen, Isha Dubey, Manuela Ciotti, Uwe Skoda, and Vivek Kumar Shukla.

None of this would have been possible without the support of my parents, Sulabha and Sanjeev Pathak, who started me on this journey when they encouraged me to pursue my interest in the social sciences and change course away from my business degree. They have seen this work develop from dissertation to manuscript, discussed ideas, commented on drafts, and aided the fieldwork. More importantly, they have been my biggest cheerleaders and earliest role models; their contributions are too numerous to enumerate. I dedicate this book to them.

1

INTRODUCTION

Contaminated Landscapes, Endocrine Disruption, and PCOS

We live in a world rife with manmade endocrine-disrupting chemicals (EDCs). These chemicals line our tins and coat our credit cards, they are the flame retardants in our mattresses and sofas, and they are in the pesticide residues we eat along with our foods, in the cosmetics we apply to our skin, and the antibacterial toothpaste we use every morning, in electronics, medical equipment, building materials, rivers and oceans, and even in the dust surrounding us. There is no escaping them. There are no longer any environments free of EDCs. We know that EDCs interfere with our hormones, but their exact consequences on health are shrouded in uncertainty. Meanwhile, every body, human or animal, tested in the last decade has shown the presence of EDCs; it is now impossible to find uncontaminated bodies to function as controls for scientific research on their effects (Bergman et al. 2013; Bushnik et al. 2010; Carpenter 2006).

What does living in the midst of such cumulative, everyday exposure mean for the health of the human population? Whereas a voice in my head says, "nothing possibly good," the lack of epidemiological data on endocrine disorder prevalence over time makes this question difficult to answer with certainty. In my field site of India—and the location where this book is set—it has become commonplace to hear complaints regarding the degraded state of health and wellness brought by "chemicals," "pollution," and the "modern." These changes are seen to have been particularly pronounced after 1991, when India embarked on a series of neoliberal economic reforms. Certainly, the country has been seeing worryingly high rates of endocrine disorders such as obesity and type II diabetes since then (Khandelwal and Reddy 2013; Wells et al. 2016). The well-documented rise in the incidence and prevalence of type II diabetes and other metabolic disorders such as heart disease in the Global South following increased engagement with globalization and industrialization has typically been blamed on shifts toward processed foods, calorie-rich diets, and decreased movement thanks to labor-saving technologies (e.g., Popkin 1993, 2001). These shifts, it is argued, lead to weight gain and obesity, which in turn lead to metabolic and endocrine issues.

DOI: 10.4324/9781003171423-1

1

Some scholars, most notably the health geographer Julie Guthman (2012), have cautioned that this is a dangerously narrow view. She argues that we have to start thinking of obesity and obesity-related disorders as complex endocrine issues that must be examined in their systemic context. This means that when it comes to obesity, we cannot think in terms of calories gained through food eaten as opposed to calories lost to energy spent through activity, with the difference between them being weight gain (or loss), alone. Rather, Guthman maintains, we must reckon with the effects of EDCs in the environment, the microbiome (the microbes within human bodies), and metabolic processes on hormonal health and dysfunction. Her ecological perspective resonates with the view taken by most of the people I spoke to and interacted with in the course of the investigations that I document in this book. Instead of focusing on calories, they blamed stress, consumer lifestyles, and a disrupted relationship between the human and the natural order for the rise in chronic health problems, including type II diabetes and heart disease.

Polycystic ovary syndrome (PCOS), whose symptoms include irregular menstruation, weight gain, cystic acne, hirsutism (excessive bodily hair), and scalp hair loss, is one of the most commonly reported endocrine disorders and the leading cause of female infertility across the globe. It is also a metabolic syndrome disorder (Ehrmann et al. 2006). Metabolic syndrome refers to a cluster of disorders that tend to co-occur and that are linked to increased risks of developing cardiovascular disease and diabetes (Eckel, Grundy, and Zimmet 2005). Generally, indices of metabolic syndrome include central obesity, high blood pressure, raised triglycerides, raised fasting glucose, and reduced HDL cholesterol. As with other metabolic syndrome disorders, PCOS is tied to obesity and increased risks of type II diabetes and coronary heart disease, and it is considered a lifestyle disease (Barber and Franks 2019; Ehrmann 2005). Although there is a dearth of epidemiological studies on the syndrome in India, public discourse and media accounts suggest that there has been a significant rise in the number of PCOS cases in the country, especially among the urban middle class, in the last two decades. For example, a 2012 article in India's leading English-language daily, *The Times of India*, states on the basis of observations of practicing gynecologists that "The number of women having PCOS has almost doubled in the last ten years" (Times of India 2012). Other news articles highlight a similar increase (e.g., Garari 2014; Khosla 2009; Nashrulla 2010; Ravichandran 2014), and medical practitioners corroborate this perceived upward trend. Of note, preliminary studies suggest that the prevalence of PCOS is much higher in India than globally. Whereas global prevalence is typically placed in the 4–11 per cent range depending upon country (Wijeyaratne, Dilini Udayangani, and Balen 2013), a study among women aged 15–24 in Mumbai placed prevalence at near 22.5 per cent or around one in four women (Joshi et al. 2014). That study was centered on young women (rather than all reproductive-aged women) of the lower socioeconomic strata, and the authors proposed that given trends in other metabolic disorders and nutritional and physical activity patterns, this prevalence might be even higher among women of the middle class.

Studies have proposed a link between PCOS and synthetic EDCs in the environment (e.g., Kandaraki et al. 2011; Palioura and Diamanti-Kandarakis 2015; Rutkowska and Rachoń 2014). However, it is difficult to establish causal links between EDCs and specific conditions. Emerging research indicates that EDCs can have significant effects at low doses but completely different types of effects at high doses (Diamanti-Kandarakis et al. 2009; Vandenberg 2014). Furthermore, the effects of EDCs are systemic, can take a long time to manifest, and are thought to be more pronounced at certain life stages (e.g., gestation, puberty). Bodies are also likely to come into contact with several EDCs in the course of a day, resulting in cumulative and interactive risk. EDCs therefore complicate notions of vulnerability, exposure, and harm. They also challenge conventional "dose determines the poison" models of toxicity which presume that some level of a toxicant can be assimilated by the body without adverse consequences (Liboiron 2016). EDCs are therefore implicated in a form of "slow violence," which Rob Nixon defines as "a violence that occurs gradually and out of sight, a violence of delayed destruction that is dispersed across time and space, an attritional violence that is typically not viewed as violence at all" (2011: 2).

There are no clear data on the types and exact volumes of various EDCs in the environment in India—or indeed the globe—or on typical exposure to EDCs of various population segments. Nevertheless, given high levels of air, water, and soil pollution in India (as I detail in a following section), it seems safe to assume that such exposure is likely to be very high, higher than in places in the Global North. Studies have consistently found that Indians carry higher body burdens—body burdens measure the accumulation of synthetic chemicals in the body—of pesticide-related EDCs than their global counterparts. The body burdens of some EDCs—such as the insecticide DDT, which has been banned across most of the world but which is still manufactured and used in India for mosquito control—have been declining with time. Nonetheless, they remain very high. Moreover, the body burdens of other insecticide-related EDCs, such as chlorpyrifos, have increased instead (Bedi et al. 2013; Bhatnagar et al. 1992). Body burden studies of EDCs in India have tended to focus on insecticide-related EDCs, and as of now, there are no clear data on the body burdens of all the myriad other EDCs to which bodies are exposed.

All this is not to say that the rise in PCOS in India should be tied to EDCs alone. As mentioned earlier, when middle-class interlocutors speak of the detrimental health effects of the "modern"—also glossed as "Westernization" or globalization—they reference 1991 as a time around which these

3

processes gained momentum. Indeed, India has been undergoing a dizzying array of changes, in both sociocultural and political–economic terms, since then. Max Liboiron, Manuel Tironi, and Nerea Calvillo (2018), in theorizing about toxicity, ask us to look beyond contamination alone to consider relations of harm; toxicity, they emphasize, is a social rather than purely chemical relation. Certain types of toxicity, in this sense, are produced by certain political–economic regimes, and they are also reproductive of these regimes. In public discourse in India, several changes after the economic liberalization of 1991 are associated with toxicity in this other sense—toxic structures and patterns of living rather than toxic matter alone. As an endocrine disorder and a lifestyle disease, PCOS is tied to both these types of toxicity. Given the ubiquity of PCOS in contemporary India and the rise in its incidence following on the heels of economic liberalization, I draw upon PCOS as lens in this book. Through PCOS, I investigate these larger issues of living amid vertiginous political–economic and sociocultural shifts and an uncertain but often viscerally felt toxicity, especially in the Global South. My focus is on the interactive biological, social, and ecological loops through which not just substances but also structures of daily life become toxic and produce harm. In particular, I argue for attention to toxic locations, that is, to locations at the interface of multiple, interacting, and cumulative pressures that are implicated in exposure to toxicity and that result in harm to health.

Polycystic Ovary Syndrome

PCOS (also known as polycystic ovary disorder, or PCOD) is named for the multiple ovarian follicles, which look like cysts, that are often found in a gynecological sonography of women with the condition. In a normal menstrual cycle, one egg is released from a dominant follicle. In PCOS, there is "follicular arrest." This means that several follicles develop simultaneously, but none reach the size required to become dominant (Soulez, Didier, and Rosenfield 1996). As a result, there may be no ovulation, and the menstrual cycle may be delayed, sporadic, or absent, leading to reduced fertility (also known as subfertility). Sometimes, menstrual cycles may be anovulatory; that is, there will be menstrual cycles without the release of an egg (Balen, Homburg, and Franks 2009; Homburg 2006).

The exact etiology, or cause, of PCOS is unknown, but both genetic predisposition and lifestyle factors are known to play a part in its development (Balen, Homburg, and Franks 2009; Ehrmann 2005). Obesity is a symptom of the condition, but it also contributes to developing PCOS and worsening other symptoms; obesity can often lead to PCOS even as PCOS often leads to obesity. Nonetheless, not all women with PCOS are obese or overweight, and the syndrome also has a "lean PCOS" phenotype. This phenotype consists of women who are not overweight and who look lean or slim and have the condition (Franks 1995).

The syndrome's name suggests that the ovaries are the focus and the major affected organs. In fact, however, PCOS, as an endocrine disorder—not just a gynecological one—is a multisystem condition with a range of diverse symptoms. These symptoms include multiple ovarian follicles, overweight or obesity, cystic acne, hirsutism (excessive bodily hair growth), scalp hair loss, insulin resistance (a precursor to diabetes in which the cells of the body become less responsive to insulin), and acanthosis nigricans (darkened skin patches resulting from insulin resistance). Symptoms such as cystic acne, male-pattern hair loss, and hirsutism (including male-pattern facial hair) are identified as resulting from excessive androgenic activity. This is the activity of hormones known as androgens, including testosterone.[1] The syndrome also brings higher risks of miscarriage, type II diabetes, and coronary heart disease (Franks 1995; Homburg 2006; Legro et al. 1999).

Not all women with PCOS will manifest all these symptoms. Importantly, not all women with PCOS present with the appearance of multiple ovarian follicles. Ovaries with such follicles are known as polycystic ovaries, and polycystic ovaries need not be an indication of PCOS either. Thus, not all women with PCOS have polycystic ovaries, and not all women with polycystic ovaries have PCOS (Balen, Homburg, and Franks 2009). Given this, diagnosis of the condition cannot rely on the presence of polycystic ovaries alone.

The Rotterdam criteria are the most commonly used criteria used to diagnose the condition. Under these criteria, a diagnosis of PCOS requires the presence of at least two of the following: (1) anovulation or irregular ovulation, (2) excess androgenic activity (as per clinical assessment on the basis of symptoms or laboratory tests), and (3) polycystic ovaries (Rotterdam ESHRE/ASRM-Sponsored PCOS Consensus Workshop Group 2004).

PCOS has no known cure. Lifestyle factors are associated with its development and manifestation, and lifestyle changes are key to its management (Balen and Rutherford 2007). Weight reduction is the primary line of management. This is the case not just for overweight or obese women but also for lean women who may have high levels of visceral fat, that is, fat near the waistline and stomach. Management also involves medication targeted at symptoms. Thus, oral contraceptives may be prescribed to regulate menstruation, ovulation inducers and reproductive technologies help combat subfertility, and insulin sensitizers aid in addressing insulin resistance and weight gain (Amsterdam ESHRE/ASRM-Sponsored 3rd PCOS Consensus Workshop Group 2012; Balen and Rutherford 2007).

Increasingly, studies have been suggesting that PCOS results from insulin resistance (Franks 1995). Some have therefore argued that PCOS has a male equivalent. Although this does not involve polycystic ovaries, it is associated with insulin resistance, central obesity, early male-pattern baldness, and other hormonal changes[2] similar to those in women (Kurzrock and Cohen 2007; Starka et al. 2005). This ties PCOS even more firmly to the metabolic syndrome and to other metabolic disorders.

The Rise of Metabolic Syndrome Disorders

Historically, South Asia recorded low levels of diabetes, hypertension, and cardiovascular risk factors. Now, though, it registers very high rates of these disorders and the metabolic syndrome. Not just incidence, but prevalence has also been increasing, especially in urban areas (Celermajer et al. 2012). In 2000, India had the highest number of people with diabetes mellitus (31.7 million). By the year 2030, that number is expected to go up to 79.4 million (Wild et al. 2004: 1051). In 2002, insulin resistance (a precursor to diabetes) as measured through surrogate markers already ranged from 20 to 55 per cent of the Indian population. The variation was attributed to population heterogeneity, with urban populations and higher socioeconomic strata showing higher rates than rural populations and lower socioeconomic strata, respectively (Misra et al. 2002; Wasir and Misra 2004). Crude estimates suggest that the prevalence of diabetes in urban populations in India is about four times that in rural populations, although rural areas are rapidly catching up (Anjana et al. 2011).

Other noncommunicable diseases are also on the rise; 53 per cent of the deaths in 2008 were attributed to such disorders (Reddy et al. 2005; Upadhyay 2012). Cardiovascular diseases accounted for 41 per cent of urban male deaths and 37 per cent of urban female deaths in India. These proportions were lower in rural areas, at 25 per cent for men and 22 per cent for women (Celermajer et al. 2012). Estimates also suggest that 20–40 per cent of the urban Indian population and 12–17 per cent of the rural population have hypertension (Khandelwal and Reddy 2013). Although detailed epidemiological evidence is lacking, there is a clear rural–urban difference in the prevalence of noncommunicable and lifestyle diseases. This difference has been tied to changes in diet and lifestyle between rural and urban areas.

Obesity and overweight are two other factors seeing an upsurge. Both tend to be higher among members of higher socioeconomic strata,[3] urban rather than rural populations, and women rather than men (Chopra et al. 2013; Kalra and Unnikrishnan 2012; Khandelwal and Reddy 2013). Between 1998 and 2016, the proportion of adult women classified as overweight or obese saw more than a twofold increase, from 9 to 21 per cent; between 2005 and 2016, the proportion of adult men classified as overweight or obese went from 11 to 19 per cent (Luhar et al. 2018). National health survey data reveal that 35.1 per cent of urban men and 47.5 per cent of urban women were overweight compared to 7.7 per cent of rural men and 11.3 per cent of rural women in 2005–2006. Furthermore, the data describe an upturn in the percentage of obese or overweight ever-married women between the ages of 15 and 49, from 11 per cent in 1998–1999 to 15 per cent in 2005–2006 (Kalra and Unnikrishnan 2012; Khandelwal and Reddy 2013). Childhood obesity is also on the rise. It went from a prevalence rate of 9.8 per cent in 2006 to 11.7 per cent in 2009 (Chopra et al. 2013).

Overall, this points to two major trends—the upswing in the burden of noncommunicable diseases in India overall and the association of this upswing with urbanization and affluence. These two trends have accelerated since the economic liberalization of India that began in 1991.

Economic Liberalization

After India gained independence from Britain in 1947, its economy was protected, production-led, and allowed for very limited consumer choice. Economic policy, influenced by a history of colonial exploitation, emphasized heavy business regulations, a large public sector, state-driven investment, and import restrictions. There had been a tentative exploration of economic reforms in the 1980s, but it was not until 1991 that a balance-of-payments crisis forced the Indian government to acquiesce to structural adjustment policies in exchange for a bailout from the International Monetary Fund. The historic economic reforms of 1991 came to mark a turning point now generally referred to as "economic liberalization" or "liberalization." In the words of then-Prime Minister P.V. Narasimha Rao, the reforms were to "convert India from ... [an] inward-looking economy into a market-friendly, outward-looking one" (quoted in Sharma 2003: 176).

Liberalization is widely considered a "watershed event for the Indian economy" (Rodrik and Subramaniam 2004: 4). Some reforms in industrial policy—such as the increased de-licensing for businesses, the tax concessions, the removal of constraints to asset buying and business expansion, and the opening up of public sector areas to the private sector—were continuations of earlier reforms. However, changes in India's external economic relations marked a clear discontinuity. Quotas restricting imports were removed, trade tariffs were decreased, the Indian rupee was devalued, restrictions on external financial transactions were eased, and foreign investment laws were liberalized (Kohli 2006). After economic liberalization, India has surfaced as one of the world's ten largest economies. India's GDP went from USD 1.096 trillion in 1991 to USD 7.16 trillion in 2015 (World Bank 2018). Indian exports went from USD 18 billion in 1990–1991 to USD 245 billion in 2010–2011, and foreign direct investment (FDI) went from USD 0.13 billion to USD 30.3 billion (Economic Times 2011). This higher per capita income also saw (and continues to see) the growth of new middle-class segments and identities.[4]

Post-Liberalization Sociocultural Transformations

As a result of the relaxation of trade tariffs, import regulations, and restrictions on businesses within India, previously inaccessible consumer products and services became much more widely available after 1991. Furthermore, economic growth and social mobility brought them within reach of consumers earlier denied such choices. A 2006 article in the *Far Eastern*

Economic Review, for example, noted that growth in discretionary shopping was driven by "upwardly mobile lower-income classes—both urban and rural—that have begun spending on a deeper and more diverse basket of basic goods" (Mahindra 2006).

A host of new aspirational media images and messages were aligned with the increased availability of goods and services. The economic reforms of 1991 more or less coincided with the introduction of satellite television in India. Prior to that, state-sponsored programming on the lone television channel, Doordarshan, focused on social concerns and social education. The satellite channels that started broadcasting after 1991, however, focused on entertainment and a more consumerist dispensation (Agrawal 1997; Mankekar 2004). They also brought international programming to India. In just five years, India went from a single television channel to a variety of 69 channels (Cullity 2002: 410). Much of the advertising and Indian programming on these channels was based on a vision of the Indian nation that was tied to consumption and to an idealized depiction of the urban middle class (Fernandes 2000a).

This coincided with a move away from the earlier national political discourse focused on development. That discourse, in which the urban middle class was largely absent, gave way to one focused on a consumption-led path to national prosperity, with a prominent, albeit idealized, urban middle class (Fernandes 2000a, 2001; Gillespie and Cheesman 2002; Rajagopal 2001). This middle class, portrayed as the face of the nation, was to negotiate India's relationship with the world through its cosmopolitan consumerism (Fernandes 2000b; Mazzarella 2003). Images in the media focused on the social and lifestyle aspirations of this class, portrayed as globally mobile and "modern-yet-Indian" (Gillespie and Cheesman 2002; Munshi 2001). Moreover, consumer lifestyles came to dominate not just advertisements (whether on TV, in magazines, or suffusing the physical landscape through billboards), but also programs on television and Bollywood movies (e.g., Dwyer 2011; Kasbekar 2006; Kohli-Khandekar 2010; Mankekar 2004; Uberoi 2001).

The increased depictions of consumer lifestyles and consumerist representations have been accompanied by an increasing acceptance of consumer culture (Mazzarella 2003; Venkatesh 1994). This is not just a function of high economic growth—Harold Wilhite (2008) points out that while overall consumer spending is highest in the South Indian state of Kerala, the state has experienced only moderate economic growth. Rather, shopping has become emblematic of a claim to a global Indianness. Ritty Lukose writes that "Increasingly, forms of consumer citizenship in the era of liberalization articulate the citizen through the notion of a right to consume, a right that must be protected through state action" (2009: 8). Other scholars of India have noted shifts in the idea of the representative citizen as a producer to that of the representative citizen as cosmopolitan consumer (Deshpande 2003; Mazzarella 2003; Vedwan 2007). Moreover, consumption in post-liberalization India is closely—if ambivalently—tied to middle-class identity. Even though members of the middle class may criticize consumer culture as debased materialism, they accept it as central to middle-class social life (van Wessel 2004). For young Indians growing up with and especially after economic liberalization, this moral ambiguity is even less of an issue (e.g., Nisbett 2007).

As with shopping, so with eating out. Once rare, eating out has progressively become integral to India's urban-centered public culture, and it is a key marker of middle classness (Fernandes 2006; Gaiha, Jha, and Kulkarni 2013). In fact, coffee shops, pizza joints, and other multinational eateries, along with shopping malls and multiplexes, form the spaces where the new urban middle classness associated with liberalization is performed, at the site of the body, through practices of consumption (McGuire 2011).

Meanwhile, the pace of life, especially for the middle class, has been affected by new communications technologies such as the mobile phone and the internet and by the restructuring of the labor market. The traditional base for middle-class jobs—public-sector employment in industries such as banking—has now shifted to the private sector, and middle-class ambition has moved away from the stability of government jobs toward employment in multinationals with expanded chances for career and salary growth (Fernandes 2000b). These jobs, however, are characterized by higher job insecurity, a need for constant adaptation, and an emphasis on efficiency. The outcome has been a move away from a middle-class work environment of job security and regular hours to a highly competitive and unstable professional environment requiring longer hours and continual improvement in productivity and skills. Although there has been an expansion in opportunities for urban middle-class women to work outside the home and an increased social acceptance of their doing so, this has often been as a result of the new financial burdens of consumption that have been placed on households. For women themselves, the effects have been uneven and contradictory:

> On the one hand, the expansion of service sector and private sector employment has produced employment opportunities for middle-class women in metropolitan centers. However, such opportunities often represent coping strategies as households attempt to negotiate increasing household costs and new lifestyle standards that correspond to public representations of the new middle class. This has produced familiar gendered pressures as middle-class women must perform a dual shift of paid and unpaid household work.
>
> (Fernandes 2000b:100–101)

Besides the increased accessibility and acceptance of employment outside the home for middle-class women, there have been other social shifts as well. While it is difficult to generalize about trends that apply equally to all of India across region, caste, socioeconomic status, community, and so on, it is nevertheless true that gender roles and performances are in flux. The Indian nation has tended to have an uneasy relationship with the project of modernity, a project associated with the uniquely European setting of the Enlightenment (Chakrabarty 2008; Chatterjee 1993). Modernity, as an ideology, celebrates individual choice, freedom from hierarchical bonds, rational thinking, scientific progress, and economic welfare (Giddens and Pierson 1998: 94). During the colonial period, modernity was seen as inherently Western, colonized India was thought to have been based on civilizational structures incompatible with modernity, and this difference was used to justify colonialism (Inden 1990; Washbrook 1997). Given this use of the project of modernity, the Indian nationalist movement looked to an updated tradition for self-definition; it would attempt to balance an engagement with modernity—which was seen as the source of the colonizer's power—with a rootedness in tradition. Gender was crucial to this balancing act (Chatterjee 1993). As a result, India's middle class has long zealously managed women's engagement with modernity as a part of a project of class distinction.

What has been novel about the period after economic liberalization, however, is the degree to which performances of the "modern" and "global" are now expected. Smitha Radhakrishnan notes:

> [there has been an] entrance of new discourses of femininity and respectability in the national mainstream. These discourses are new in that they center around a "new" liberal Indian woman who embraces a high-tech education, and stands up against such "traditional" practices as dowry, conventionally accepted as an inevitable ill of Indian society.
>
> (2009: 196)

Radhakrishnan adds,

> The important thread running through all the narratives women articulate is the idea of the "right" amount of freedom—not as much as abroad, where your sexual and leisure behaviors might indicate a rejection of family, and thus, a loss of culture, but not so little freedom as in either an earlier Indian generation, or, implicitly, those less educated and less well-off Indians who cannot exercise these freedoms.
>
> (2009: 207)

What constitutes a "good balance" between the traditional and the modern, then, has shifted considerably toward the modern for the urban middle class (Gilbertson 2014a). Professional women have come to occupy an important

10

social, economic, and symbolic position in India, and the public visibility of women and their freedom to pursue careers is now considered central to the identity of the professional segment of the middle class (Ganguly–Scrase 2003). Furthermore, educational achievements and professional status are not just important to a woman's career, but they now bring improved marriage prospects (Radhakrishnan 2011; Sharangpani 2010). Nevertheless, these new opportunities have not displaced conventional responsibilities, and women are still deemed responsible for child-rearing and household management.

Contaminated Landscapes

Post-liberalization changes have extended beyond these economic and sociocultural realms; accelerated urbanization and industrialization have had far-reaching implications in terms of environmental indices. In a Pew Research Center study from 2007, 79 per cent of Indians felt that pollution was a "very big problem" (Economist 2008). This concern is not without cause. The removal of trade restrictions saw greater inflow of foreign direct investment into the polluting sectors of the economy than into nonpolluting ones; these sectors also saw exports grow (Gamper-Rabindran and Jha 2004). In 2019, India was reported to be the country with the fifth most polluted air (IQ*Air* 2020b). The Indian city of Ghaziabad was ranked as the city with the most polluted air in 2019, and 10 of the 15 most polluted cities in the world are located in India (IQ*Air* 2020a). A World Bank report found that there had been large relative increases in particulate matter in air in India from 1990 to 2013, and it estimated that such air pollution costs India about 8.5 per cent of its GDP (World Bank Group and Institute for Health Metrics and Evaluation 2016). A rise in the number of coal-fired plants, construction projects, and cars has been blamed for this state of affairs (Harris 2014). In particular, the transport sector is a major culprit—government subsidies encourage the use of the more polluting diesel over gasoline in vehicles (Pearson and Katakey 2014). Meanwhile, the number of construction projects and cars on Indian roads are constantly increasing as the economy grows. Emissions standards for vehicles are comparatively lax, and vehicles sold in India lag anywhere from 7 to 12 years behind Europe's emissions standards (H.T. Correspondents 2013). The impact of this on human life is staggering—estimates place the burden of outdoor air pollution at 620,000 premature deaths per year; this is equivalent to the loss of 650 million years of life just for those living in urban areas (Greenstone and Pande 2014). This is before even considering the consequences for wellness and quality of life. Besides being linked to respiratory diseases, air pollution can also lead to EDC exposure. Inhalation is one of the multiple routes of bodily exposure to EDCs, and exposure to air pollution has been tied to fertility and reproductive issues (Carré et al. 2017; Conforti et al. 2018; Darbre 2018).

Water pollution is another major concern. From 1993 to 2005, water pollution levels have more than doubled, and the upward trend continues. India has three out of the ten rivers that are estimated to drain up to 90 per cent of plastic waste into the oceans—the Ganges, the Meghna-Brahmaputra, and the Indus (Schmidt, Krauth, and Wagner 2017). Added to this, ineffective waste water treatment and poorly implemented environmental regulations result in industrial and household waste entering waterways and, from there, ecologies. Up to 80 per cent of India's urban waste, including industrial effluent and sewage, ends up in rivers, and the problem has been getting worse as a result of the urban growth that has been accompanying economic development (Pepper 2007; Singh et al. 2018). Water pollution is not just a problem in terms of India's rivers—pesticides, EDCs, heavy metals, and medicines such as antibiotics find their way underground into the water table, even into bottled water, and from there, into the bodies of Indians (Agrawal, Pandey, and Sharma 2010).

India is heavily dependent upon pesticides and insecticides (known sources of EDCs) for agriculture. The reliance on pesticides has only increased with time: where the total use was 154 metric tons in 1954, it was 88,000 metric tons in 2000—an increase of 570 per cent in less than 50 years (Mathur et al. 2005). Moreover, guidelines regarding pesticide use are not stringently implemented, many farmers are unaware of maximum use limits, and banned pesticides continue to be used. In short, pesticide use in the country is excessive. As a result, pesticide residues on crops, produce and food, and in the air, soil, and water can be extremely high (Chakraborty et al. 2017; Gupta 2004; Hashmi et al. 2020; Srivastava et al. 2011; Yadav et al. 2015). The presence of pesticide residues means the presence of EDCs, and samples from waterways across the country show the presence of multiple such pesticide-related EDCs (e.g., Sankararamakrishnan, Kumar Sharma, and Sanghi 2005; Singare 2016; Tiwari, Sahu, and Pandit 2016).

Women in contemporary urban India find themselves having to navigate this pervasive pollution and geographies rife with EDCs while also learning to live with the new consumer imperatives, changing gender norms, and much more demanding work structures that have followed liberalization. Simultaneously, urban middle-class Indian women face high rates of PCOS, higher than global averages and higher than those faced by women of earlier generations. Through its effects on appearance and fertility, PCOS poses risks to women's marriageability and to their conventional roles as wives and mothers. An extant literature on India highlights how childlessness and fertility issues are highly stigmatized for women, regardless of life stage or class status (Inhorn and Bharadwaj 2007; Jeffery, Jeffery, and Lyon 1989; Mehta and Kapadia 2008; Riessman 2000). Thus, the widespread and ubiquitous nature of PCOS in India, combined with its potential to disrupt normative feminine sociocultural biographies, makes this a particularly salient condition in the lives of Indian women.

The Field Site and Methods

When I first arrived in India for what would become this study, I was not interested in examining PCOS; I had planned to explore changing health-related and bodily practices in post-liberalization India. I have PCOS myself. I was diagnosed—in India, no less—at the age of 27. The condition, however, never preoccupied me much. I was certainly not looking to study it or, as an Indian woman with the condition, to be the subject of my own investigation. During my exploratory fieldwork, however, the topic of PCOS kept coming up; I read about it in newspapers, heard about it in conversations, and met women with the condition until I felt I could not ignore the condition. Ultimately, it became the focus of this project.

The book is based on long-term ethnographic fieldwork carried out from 2012 to 2015 and then again in 2016 and 2017. The research was based in Mumbai, which is not just the capital of the state of Maharashtra, but also India's financial, commercial, and entertainment capital. Mumbai is the richest city in South Asia. In addition, it is the region's only alpha world city—a city linking a major economic region with the global economy (Globalization and World Cities Network 2012). The city also houses India's largest movie industry, Bollywood. As such, Mumbai looms large in the national imagination, and scholars of South Asia have noted how Mumbai functions as a subject for a modern cosmopolitan imaginary of India and an imaginary of a specifically Indian modernity (Hansen 2001; Mazzarella 2003; Patel 2004; Rao 2006).

Within Mumbai, my focus was on the urban middle class, which is portrayed as being the most affected by rising rates of PCOS. This is also the class whose lifestyles are depicted as the aspirational ideal in the media and in public discourse and which "sets the terms of reference of Indian society" (Jaffrelot and Van der Veer 2008: 19). Middle classness in India is, however, a notoriously difficult category to pin down. As William Mazzarella observed,

> Even if we accept the validity of the middle class descriptor for India, we are still left with a sense that the term is being stretched to cover a staggering diversity of socio-economic and cultural situations. An income that in smaller towns or rural areas might qualify a family as middle class will, in the major Indian cities, only be barely enough to sustain life outside the slums. Nor is income alone a reliable index to middle class status even within urban contexts. A Bombay survey of the 1990s reported that schoolteachers bringing home Rs. 1200/month considered themselves middle class while factory workers earning three times that amount identified themselves as working class.
>
> (2005: 2–3)

13

As a result of this complexity, scholars tend to see middle classness in India as a performative socioeconomic grouping rather than an economic classification (e.g., Deshpande 2003; Donner and de Neve 2011; Fernandes 2006; Mazzarella 2005). Claims to middle classness tend to ignore caste divisions and focus on English education and the professional employment it bestows, even though education and professional employment are themselves linked to higher caste status. Moreover, "a range of representational practices centered around particular characteristics of consumption, style, and social distinction" (Fernandes 2006: 141) are central to middle-class status. Within the larger middle class, Fernandes and Heller (2006) have outlined three major segments: the professional middle class bearing professional educational credentials; a petit bourgeoisie consisting of merchants and shopkeepers that attempts to emulate the professional middle class; and an educated segment concentrated in nonprofessional, lower ranking jobs. My focus was on the urban professional middle class (including members of "business"—petit bourgeoisie—families with professional qualifications, i.e., those shifting into the professional middle class) in Mumbai. This segment was dominated by English-speaking, upwardly mobile members with aspirational consumption patterns who benefited from the opportunities brought by liberalization, and their status was reflected in lifestyles that involved comfort with English, knowledge of global (usually American) popular culture, engagement with and economic access to new practices of consumption, and at least an undergraduate English-language education with potential for professional white-collar employment. Through their engagement with global popular culture and consumption patterns and their reflexive awareness of themselves in relation to the world, members of this class could also be seen to be displaying a "cosmopolitan disposition" (Skrbis, Kendall, and Woodward 2004: 117).

The study involved a total of 154 participants. The core ethnography presented in this book is drawn from in-depth interviews, informal conversations, and long-term observations across social settings of 30 professional middle-class women over the age of 21, resident in Mumbai, and possessing a medical diagnosis of PCOS. These women all satisfied the performative criteria associated with professional middle-class status listed earlier. Care was taken to ensure that the they were not drawn only from certain communities (interlocutors included, for example, Kashmiris, Punjabis, Bengalis, Gujaratis, Maharashtrians, Mangaloreans, and Tamilians, among others), religions (the core group included Christians, Hindus, Muslims, Jains, and Parsis), or locales in Mumbai. Given the centrality of concerns related to marriage and motherhood to women's lives in India, of these 30 women, 10 were never married, 10 were married without children, and 10 were married with children. Although initially women were chosen to fall within these categories, given the extended nature of the fieldwork, some interlocutors shifted categories and life stages (that is, some got married, gave birth, or got divorced) during that time.

I am an Indian citizen who has lived abroad for almost as many years as I have lived in India. I largely came of age in India around the time of economic liberalization, and I remember the heady initial days of satellite television and new consumer goods coming to the country. Since then, I have been based mostly outside of India, although I have family in Mumbai, and I visit often and for extended periods of time. As such, I occupy a liminal space as a simultaneous insider and outsider, which has enabled the building of rapport through shared experiences with my interlocutors while also allowing me to ask about India-specific experiences that I am not expected to recognize. I also have an extensive social network in Mumbai.

I identified the core interlocutors with PCOS for this study through referrals from within that social network. This allowed for triangulation of the data gathered from interviews with the data gleaned from observations of interlocutors and their practices in naturalistic and social settings. The core interlocutors varied in their ages (spanning the ages 22–45), PCOS symptoms, therapeutic itineraries, religious/community backgrounds, and household composition (nuclear, extended nuclear). Not all these women were actively undergoing treatment for their PCOS; some were on medication for some symptoms, others had made or would sporadically attempt lifestyle changes to manage the condition, and yet others were living with their symptoms without undertaking interventions.

The core material was supplemented by a media analysis of articles on PCOS and interviews with lay interlocutors, medical professionals, and the husbands of women with PCOS in order to understand public perceptions of and public discourses regarding PCOS, its etiology, and its relationship to other chronic metabolic disorders. The media analysis was centered on the English-language print media, which is the media favored by the urban professional middle class. Articles (42 total) from the decade 2005–2014 were chosen through keyword searches for the terms "PCOS," "PCOD," "hormonal disorder," "hormonal imbalance," and "menstrual disorder."

The supplemental interviews were conducted with (a) lay professional middle-class interlocutors (those who did not have the condition; n = 30), (b) healthcare professionals involved in the diagnosis or management of the syndrome (n = 30), and (c) husbands of women with PCOS (n = 10). The sample of lay interlocutors spanned two age ranges: 21–35 (n = 15; 10 women, 5 men) and 36–50 (n = 15; 10 women, 5 men). This allowed for a sampling of opinions across genders and across the generational divide of those that came of age prior to economic liberalization and those that came of age during and after it. Interviews with key interlocutors and preliminary fieldwork suggested that dermatologists, gynecologists, endocrinologists, dietitians/nutritionists, homeopaths, and Ayurvedic practitioners were the healthcare professionals most involved in diagnosing and managing PCOS. I therefore interviewed five of each of these types of practitioners, all practicing in Mumbai. Interviews were conducted at the practitioners' places of work, and given practitioners' hectic schedules, interviews were frequently delayed or halted and resumed later (if patients arrived or consultations were to start). As a result, I often spent several hours in consulting rooms, clinics, and hospitals observing patient concerns and interactions. In the case of the husbands of women with PCOS, I typically spoke to the women prior to interviewing their spouses. After that, if the husbands were amenable, I interviewed them alone. If not, they were interviewed in the presence of their wives. Interviews were typically conducted in coffee shops or in interlocutors' homes.

I drew from my own experiences with PCOS to build rapport and guide me to themes for research, and I observed reactions to my self-disclosure to gauge how the condition was responded to, stigmatized, hidden, or talked about. Besides this, I engaged in long-term observation of professional middle-class interactions and conversations in Mumbai and conducted interviews with key interlocutors and among professional middle-class interlocutors (n = 54) to understand bodily practices, work and domestic routines, and lifestyles among this class. Given the professional middle-class segment's comfort with English, interviews were primarily conducted in that language, although code switching between English, Hindi, and sometimes Marathi was common. In rare cases where entire quotes were in Hindi or Marathi, only the translations have been provided; in most cases, however, quotes are presented to include words or phrases in Hindi and Marathi along with translations. The research was approved by the University of Arizona's Institutional Review Board, informed consent was obtained from all study participants, and all interlocutor names are pseudonyms unless mentioned otherwise.

Living amid Toxicity

Processes of and battles over rendering toxicity knowable and perceptible (or imperceptible) and the politics of uncertainty involved in these processes have come under growing scrutiny within science and technology studies (e.g., Fortun and Fortun 2005; Murphy 2006; Nash 2006; Wylie 2018). Some of these studies have also examined these issues as they pertain to EDCs (Frickel 2004; Langston 2010; Liboiron 2016; Vogel 2012). At the same time, a rich body of literature within—and at the junctures of—medical and environmental anthropology has examined toxic exposures and asked what it means to live in the midst of toxicity (e.g., Checker 2007; Geissler and Prince 2020; Kannuri and Jadhav 2018; Nading 2020; Roberts 2017; Shapiro 2015; Tironi 2018). This literature points out that there is no escaping the toxic world; the proliferation of manmade industrial substances has also brought the proliferation of manmade toxicants. Some—that is, the marginalized and the vulnerable—are less able to escape toxicity than others, but all of us are affected. We cannot return to a purer, untainted, uncontaminated world. Rather than focusing on particular substances, studies within this tradition therefore examine efforts to engage with toxic encounters in the course of creating lives deemed to be worth living. The anthropologist Alex Nading (2020) calls this dynamic of being affected by toxicity while also learning to affect in return "toxic worlding."

This book revolves around the toxic worlding of urban professional middle-class Indian women with PCOS as they navigate their toxic location—and both the harms and the pleasures that this location brings—that renders them vulnerable to the condition. The focus on women within this class, which can be considered a relatively elite class within India, is not to suggest that the burdens placed on urban middle-class women are higher than those placed on women from other socioeconomic strata (especially from low-income groups) or to imply that these women do not occupy a position of comparative privilege. Rather, I focus on women within this class for their position at the confluence of several structural factors that render them vulnerable despite—and even as a result of—their seemingly elite status. In the chapters that follow, I explore two main themes: (1) how toxic locations within sociocultural, political–economic, and political–ecological structures are implicated in endocrine disorders such as PCOS, and (2) how the biosocial disruptions caused by PCOS are affecting and being acted upon by women, reflecting changes in urban middle-class life in India. Chapter 2 centers on public discourses about PCOS and the critique contained within them of an emerging relationship between the body and its environment that is seen as characteristically modern, toxic, and implicated in the rise of metabolic disorders. These discourses reveal how environmental and sociocultural determinants of health in middle-class India are being transformed by an accelerated engagement with consumer globalization. In Chapter 3, these changing determinants of health are linked to the mounting structural burdens placed on urban professional middle-class Indian women throughout their life course. These structural burdens interact with Indians' susceptibility to metabolic disorders to result in toxic environments that compromise women's wellbeing and result in harm through conditions such as PCOS. Chapter 4 examines how women make decisions about which practitioners to consult and what treatments to seek to manage their condition. It chronicles the typical diagnostic and therapeutic itineraries of women with the condition and details different medical and paramedical practitioners' views of the syndrome and of the syndrome's relationship to a toxic environment. The chapter also considers how interactions between medical practitioners and women with PCOS reflect new realities of health and healthcare in India, and how they can present barriers to women's management of the condition. Chapter 5 and Chapter 6 are dedicated to women's lived experiences of PCOS. These lived experiences become a lens into the commodification of health in India and into new middle-class subjectivities linked to reasonings of risk and probability in Chapter 5. Women's attention to symptoms and risks forms a limited resource which interacts with assessments of significance at various life stages, foregrounding certain concerns while others become less immediate, and affecting embodied experiences of the condition. Meanwhile, new medical technologies allow the future to be thought of in terms of probabilities and to be imagined in medicalized terms, mitigating the social risks of symptoms such as subfertility. Chapter 6 revolves around intimate modernities and emerging conceptions of family. A comparatively limited concern with childbearing forms a part of women's self-representations as members of the urban professional middle class; "modern-yet-Indian" gender norms in this class allow women to define themselves through their educational and professional qualifications (even when not working outside the home) rather than through their roles in the private sphere. These attitudes to fertility are further enabled by ideals of companionate marriage, as women privilege companionship over fertility and negotiate expectations regarding family size and marital priorities with their partners. Women's conjugal expectations and experiences also shed light on an emerging form of "supportive" masculinity.

Overall, the book describes how PCOS is a toxicity-related disruption to urban professional middle-class women's lives and to conventional feminine biographies centered on marriage and childbearing. Nevertheless, many of the post-liberalization political–economic changes linked to the toxic locations that render women vulnerable to PCOS also provide the potential for new "modern" gender, conjugal, and family norms that urban professional middle-class women can draw upon to negotiate different identities and aspirations for themselves. Women's lived experiences are a testament not just to the harms of toxicity but also to the pleasures that toxic structures can bring and to resilience in the face of their harms. My interlocutors negotiated relationships with healthcare practitioners and partners through their PCOS, grappled with the condition as it interacted with their aspirations, and engaged with their symptoms and risks sometimes with resignation and apathy, rarely with despair, and often with humor and grace. In the pages that follow, I aim to do their richly textured experiences, their narratives, and their voices justice.

Notes

1 Androgens are often termed "male hormones." This is, however, simplistic and misleading, as androgens are present across sexes, although at different levels and in different proportions in relation to other hormones.
2 Lower levels of follicle stimulating hormone and sexual hormone binding globulin and higher free androgens.
3 This is in direct contrast to trends in countries such as the United States and Israel, where overweight and obesity are associated with lower socioeconomic indicators. In India, obesity and overweight have been associated with sedentary lifestyles—which are more common among the higher socioeconomic strata—as well as calorie-rich diets. Individuals in the higher socioeconomic strata tend to be more removed from physical labor, engage in less activity thanks to labor-saving devices and domestic staff, and have access to more food and diets high in fats, oils, and simple carbohydrates. However, there is some evidence that economic growth and the proliferation of processed foods among low-income

groups, combined with rising concerns regarding obesity-related noncommunicable diseases and exposure to global, slimmer body ideals among the higher
socioeconomic strata, are resulting in changes to these patterns.

4 There is a lot of controversy over defining poverty rates in India, although poverty is generally thought to have declined after economic liberalization. Data
from the United Nations Development Program indicate that the global hunger
index for India went from 30.4 per cent in 1988–1992 to 23.7 per cent in 2004–
2009, and the poverty headcount ratio went from 37.2 per cent in 2004–2005
to 29.8 in 2009–2010 (United Nations Development Programme 2011). This
is in spite of the fact that being classified as "below the poverty line" in India
brings significant benefits to those who can qualify.

2

"A NEW NORMAL"

Health Since Economic Liberalization

All through my time in Mumbai as I conducted fieldwork for this project on PCOS (and even these days, as I study other health-related dimensions), I was privy to the constant lament that people were no longer concerned about their health. Typically, this frustrated chorus came from those over the age of 35. It had, however, almost achieved the status of accepted wisdom, such that I even heard the sentiment echoed by those who were younger. Such laments would usually come up unsolicited when talking about the habits of the young (that is, people under the age of around 35) or when referencing the rise in the so-called "lifestyle diseases" in post-liberalization India. While there may have been some generational nostalgia that was rendering the past in rose-tinted shades at play here, such observations were also referencing the dramatic shifts in population health that India has experienced in the last couple of decades. As mentioned in Chapter 1, data show that although India has seen a decline in mortality and infectious diseases, there has been a sharp and perceptible rise in chronic diseases, especially the metabolic syndrome disorders of type II diabetes and coronary heart disease, since the economic liberalization of the country (Celermajer et al. 2012; Griffiths and Bentley 2001; Khandelwal and Reddy 2013; Misra and Khurana 2008; Shetty 2002; Wasir and Misra 2004). Not only are cases growing, but prevalence is also high; the incidence of type II diabetes is at epidemic proportions, and India is now known as the "diabetes capital of the world" (Wells et al. 2016).

Within public health, the shift toward higher rates of metabolic syndrome disorders that follows increasing development and closer engagement with processes of globalization is widely recognized as the "nutrition transition" (Popkin 1993). The nutrition transition conceptualizes such a rise in metabolic syndrome disorders as a result of reduced movement and the increased consumption of calorie-dense foods. It is premised upon an "energy balance" or "calories in, calories out" model that assumes that the difference between caloric—or energy—input (through food intake) and caloric expenditure (through physical activity) results in the bodily storage of fat, which is reflected in weight gain or loss. However, in the comments I was hearing in Mumbai, it was not reduced movement and increased food

DOI: 10.4324/9781003171423-2

intake that was being blamed for the purported reduction in physical well-being since economic liberalization. Instead, I would hear about stress, disrupted meal and sleep times, eating out, and pollution.

Medical anthropologists have long noted that lay discourses on health and medical conditions can function as metamedical commentary on sociopolitical dimensions within a society (e.g., Farmer 1988; Nichter 2001). For example, Arthur Kleinman (1986) has detailed how in China, memories of political violence from the Cultural Revolution were incorporated into bodily symptoms and termed neurasthenia. Speaking about neurasthenia became a way for people to speak of the suffering that resulted from this political violence. Talking about bodily health is therefore a way to talk about the health of a society, community, and polity. As Byron Good pointed out in his seminal article on medical semantics:

> The meaning of a disease category cannot be understood simply as a set of defining symptoms. It is rather a "syndrome" of typical experiences, a set of words, experiences, and feelings which typically "run together" for the members of a society. Such a syndrome is not merely a reflection of symptoms linked with each other in natural reality, but a set of experiences associated through networks of meaning and social interaction in a society. This conception of medical semantics directs our attention to the use of medical discourse to articulate the experience of distinctive patterns of social stress, to the use of illness language to negotiate relief for the sufferer, and thus to the constitution of the meaning of medical language in its use in a variety of communicative contexts.
>
> (1977: 27)

The sociocultural construction of a disease and the categories that get associated with that disease hence go beyond the biological. They speak to the socioeconomic and the sociopolitical, indexing wider social conditions. Similarly, individuals draw up their own schemas, different from those of medical experts, regarding health conditions and their own risks of those conditions. They base these schemas on observations of cases among their networks, observations of cases of those in the public eye, and formal and informal sources of information, such as news media and medical professionals (Davison, Smith, and Frankel 1991). This "lay epidemiology" is a collective, rather than an individual, enterprise, and it involves discussion and corroboration among social networks. Although lay epidemiology draws from discourses from the formal medical and scientific community, it is not entirely congruent with or in agreement with these more technocratic discourses. Overall then, public discourses about health conditions, as metamedical commentary and as lay epidemiology, point to lived experiences of those conditions, subjective assessments of risk, lay perceptions of causality related to disorders, and wider biosocial stressors prevalent in a society.

21

Taking public discourses about a lack of care in nurturing physical well-being and about the profusion of lifestyle disorders in India after economic liberalization seriously therefore has the potential to illuminate public perceptions regarding shifts related to health. Perhaps more importantly, these public discourses can lead us to overlooked transformations in lifestyles—beyond recognized and documented changes in physical activity and diet—that affect experiences of health and wellness. In the case of India, PCOS lends itself to metamedical commentary because of its links not just to other noticeably increasing metabolic and lifestyle disorders but also to menstrual issues, which have special significance in local conceptions of health.

Indian popular health culture is heavily influenced by frameworks of "indigenous" alternative or complementary medicine, such as Ayurveda, Unani, and homeopathy,[1] and people regularly mix therapies from these systems with biomedical treatments (Halliburton 2004). These indigenous systems are premised upon ecological frameworks that treat the body as a microcosm of its universe (e.g., Gold 1998; Leslie 1996; Nichter 2001). The body is thought to be responsive to degeneration in the sociopolitical, economic, and environmental realms, and, in turn, an afflicted body contributes to the degeneration of these realms. Bodily rhythms, such as those of hunger, digestion, defecation, sleep, and menstruation, are highly esteemed by these ecological models. Moreover, abnormalities in bodily cycles are seen as indicative of affliction (Bode 2008; Nichter 1981; Zimmermann 1980). Menstrual cycles are considered particularly important indices of wellness, and their regularity—or lack thereof—is thought to signal not just the state of the health of individual women but also of the health of the social body and the body politic.

Given the significance placed upon menstrual irregularities (one of the most common symptoms of PCOS) in local conceptions of health, the links between PCOS and other metabolic syndrome disorders that are on the rise in India, and the ubiquity of the syndrome, in this chapter, I use PCOS to engage with public discourses about changes in health, wellness, and conceptions of the body after the economic liberalization of India. Such discourses reference wide-ranging transformations in environmental and sociocultural determinants of health and provide insights into how new regimes of production and consumption are reflected in new ways of treating the body. They also reveal a critique of an emerging relationship between the body and its environment that is seen as characteristically modern, toxic, and implicated in the rise of metabolic disorders such as PCOS.

PCOS in the Media

To understand public discourses about PCOS, it is important to understand how the condition is portrayed in the media. To examine how the news media were depicting PCOS, I therefore conducted a close reading of news pieces that discussed the syndrome. My investigation was centered

22

on the English-language print media, as this was the media favored by the urban middle class, which is most likely to experience high rates of PCOS. Samples were chosen using keyword searches for "PCOS," "PCOD," "hormonal disorder," "hormonal imbalance," and "menstrual disorder" from the period January 2005 to June 2014. The search yielded 42 articles from the seven leading national English-language newspapers, *The Times of India*, *Hindustan Times*, *Indian Express*, *DNA*, *Hindu*, *Mumbai Mirror*, and *Asian Age*, and one news magazine, *India Today*.

The media samples all described PCOS as widespread in urban India. One article highlighted a higher prevalence in India than worldwide: "Internationally, one in ten women suffers from PCOS. In India, experts estimate it to be one in five" (Nashrulla 2010). Another mentioned a similar prevalence of one in five women in India, whereas six articles placed it higher, in the 30–35 per cent range. Furthermore, news articles stated that PCOS was "on the rise" (Khosla 2009; Mukerjee 2012; Ravichandran 2014; Times of India 2012), that there was "growing prevalence" (Nashrulla 2010), and that PCOS cases had seen an "alarming rise" (Kumar 2007) or "increase in the number" (Garari 2014). Many quoted gynecologists who highlighted this rise in prevalence: "Incidents of PCOD have increased from 5% to 20% among adolescent girls over the last five to eight years" (Majumdar 2010), "The number of women having PCOS has almost doubled in the last ten years" (Times of India 2012), and "Although it existed 15 years ago as well, in recent years, incidence of PCOD have [sic] increased almost two-to-three fold" (Suryanarayan 2007).

This rise was linked to several factors. Whereas a few articles assigned partial responsibility to heightened awareness and improved diagnostic technologies, the more recurring motif was of modernity and its consequences. One article in *The Times of India* featured the title "Modern lifestyle increases PCOS cases" (2012) and suggested that the "problem is serious among the affluent class." It did not elaborate upon what exactly a modern lifestyle entailed, why such a lifestyle was having adverse consequences on the endocrine system, or why PCOS was more pronounced among the affluent. "Modern food habits" came under scrutiny in one article (Majumdar 2010), and two mentioned "irregular eating" times (Nashrulla 2010). Still others spoke of changes in lifestyles and food habits, especially junk food and sedentary lifestyles. Many pieces linked PCOS to obesity, pointing to weight gain as causative.

Stress was a major feature, considered to be characteristic of modern lifestyles, that was highlighted. Articles asserted that "The reasons [for the rise in PCOS]—high stress and poor lifestyle choices—are characteristic of a generation on the fast track" (Nashrulla 2010) or "Our fast-paced lifestyle worsens the condition, forcing it to manifest early in life" (Pal 2013). Other stressors included the "stress of the studies and occupation" (Gouri 2012) or the pressures of examinations and jobs involving tight deadlines and long commutes. Sleep patterns also came under scrutiny, with articles either suggesting that irregular and insufficient sleep increased the chances of developing PCOS or with them recommending longer and more regular sleep cycles to manage the condition. Finally, four articles pointed to pollutants, including the ingestion of pesticides and adulterated food, as contributory factors.

On the whole, PCOS was depicted in these media samples as an ailment associated with modernity and contemporary life. The articles presented junk food, a lack of movement, and stress as the norm, but they didn't really explain how these hectic "modern" lifestyles, stress, or pollution were implicated in endocrine disturbances. Instead, they emphasized modern living as stressful, rife with the adverse effects of environmental degradation, and antithetical to wellbeing, and they seemed to assume that readers would understand how and why these aspects were inherently unhealthy.

A Lay Epidemiology of PCOS

Although there were several overlaps between the representations of PCOS in the media and lay perceptions of the condition, there were also important differences. To explore the lay epidemiology of PCOS in Mumbai, I had conducted in-depth semi-structured interviews with a purposive sample of 30 professional middle-class interlocutors who were resident in Mumbai. This sample included women and men who did not have PCOS and who were not medical professionals. This allowed for perceptions unaffected by medical training or personal, lived experience. Interlocutors spanned two age ranges: 21–35 (n = 15; 10 women, 5 men) and 36–65 (n = 15; 10 women, 5 men) to sample for opinions from members of generations that came of age before as well as after economic liberalization. Although women formed the bulk of those interviewed, I also interviewed men to understand how the condition was viewed across gender lines.

Most interlocutors echoed the media samples in their contention that there had been a rise in PCOS prevalence. Male interlocutors were in general less voluble on the subject, given that PCOS was perceived as a women's health issue, but otherwise, there were no notable patterns of difference across interlocutor groups (i.e., across age and gender categories). When I asked about factors leading to this rise, I received general health- and lifestyle-related observations rather than specific routes of causation. The responses did, however, yield some key semantic themes and fields of association (see Table 2.1 for an overview of themes): those of defective modernization, the disruption of the natural order, and the difficulties in balancing the traditional and the modern.

Defective Modernization and Stress

As in the media samples, interlocutors described a "defective modernization" (Nichter 2001; Simonelli 1987) that was harming people's physical wellbeing. Such defective modernization was characterized by highly

Table 2.1 Themes in Interviews about Women's Chronic Health Issues

Theme	Women over 36	Women under 35	Men over 36	Men under 35	Total
Total	10	10	5	5	30
Stress	10	5	4	3	22
Diet	7	4	4	1	16
Exercise	2	4	3	1	10
Pollution/adulterants	5	1	2	2	10
Meal timings	3	1	1	-	5
Sleep/lack of routine	2	2	-	-	4
Medicines	3	-	1	-	4

stressful jobs, new pressures of consumption, and a demand for quick fixes and immediate results. Geeta, a homemaker with grown children, had a view echoed by many: "These days, it has become very competitive. Even at the school level ... stress level is very high." College professor Leela spoke of highly competitive work and educational environments that were resulting in amplified stress levels. Shefali, a communications professional, brought up the changing nature of work:

> Stress levels are going up. Working style is becoming more hectic; time-to-time—we are working all the time. Work is going with you, even on leave, with smartphones and email.

Arun, working in insurance, also blamed smartphones, which allowed work to intrude into nonwork hours, and the information technology and business process outsourcing culture of working according to the time schedules of the United States or elsewhere while living in India. He also highlighted other changes in work structures:

> Life has become too hectic. Before it was an eight-hour working day—now it is 12 hours for everything. Travelling is 3–4 hours both ways.... There is no time for personal hobbies.

Thirty-one-year-old Krishna, a finance professional, echoed these comments. He also spoke of the stress caused by a hectic urban lifestyle, which included long commutes that made managing PCOS difficult.

A 61-year-old homemaker, Manju, connected tension—a term commonly used to reference stress in India (e.g., Halliburton 2005; Mendenhall et al. 2012)—to women's hormones and periods:

> Periods are unbalanced, hormones are changing, their pattern of life—there is tension, anxiety. Sometimes it is genetic also, but nowadays it has become more because of the tension and anxiety.

They are bleeding more, or not bleeding at all, bleeding early, stopping early also. And even the main bleeding cycle of 4–5 days is reducing.

When asked to elaborate regarding this tension, Manju could not offer specifics. She could only say again, "tension and anxiety is so much, so much. For every small thing the tension is there." Sheetal, in her 50s, also spoke of more general stress: "We don't live a very peaceful life these days. Constantly there is a struggle for something." Others elaborated on this constant striving as being related to the consumer culture that had resulted from India's closer engagement with consumer globalization. Prachi mentioned urban households being "constantly exposed to new things [consumer goods]" which led to relentless financial pressures. Leela agreed: "There is also this competition that what their friends have, they want." She felt that consumer pressures contributed to high levels of stress, which went on to contribute to PCOS. As a college professor, she regularly interacted with young adults (her students) and young female colleagues in their 30s, and she believed that hormonal irregularities were much more common than they had been a couple of decades prior.

Defective modernization was also linked to a growing reliance on "outside food." Prachi's contention that "*Ghar ka khaana* [home-cooked food] is best" was oft repeated, and interlocutors blamed increased eating out and the consumption of foods such as pizzas, burgers, Maggi (noodles), and *wada pao* (fried potato patty sandwiched in white bread) for metabolic disorders. Even when referencing these changes in diet, however, interlocutors did so largely through reference to stress and time pressures. For example, Farhana unfavorably compared contemporary food choices with those of an earlier generation, mentioning taste preferences along with a paucity of time:

> We end up eating junk food. Our grandmothers and mothers— bread they would not even consider as a food. It was always *roti*. Now, we only want bread for breakfast. There is no time to make *roti*s.

Hemant, from among the male interlocutors under the age of 35, felt that contemporary urban life meant "No time to eat. More likely to eat junk food … more accessible … you can sit in the house and call for it [to be delivered]." Here, it is worth mentioning that my interlocutors focused on food that was not cooked within the home. As interlocutors saw it, the problem was not calorie-dense home-cooked meals but rather new practices of frequent eating out, takeaway, or meal deliveries.

Interlocutor views followed a similar trend, that of implicating stress and hectic schedules, when referencing reduced physical activity. For example, 27-year-old journalist Milind blamed a rise in desk jobs and sedentary lifestyles for a drop in physical activity. He added that hectic schedules then made it difficult to fit in required levels of movement. Two other male interlocutors also mentioned the lack of time to exercise. Unhealthy food and physical activity patterns were seen to result from the stress of urban living. However, interlocutors stated that while taking to these negative "modern" practices, Indians had not adopted other, more positive aspects of modernity, such as "exercise culture." The insurance professional mentioned earlier, Arun, spoke of faulty dietary patterns and exercise issues as intertwined:

> Diet has changed. We have adopted Western culture totally. Problem is, we don't work as hard as Americans. There is no exercise culture.

This was reiterated by Priyanka, who commented that exercise was "not part of our culture."

Disruption of the Natural Order

For my interlocutors, the body with PCOS was also emblematic of post-liberalization India's disordered relationship with a natural order. This was indexed through mentions to bodily rhythms and the degradation of the environment. Irregular or improper meal times were deemed causative factors when it came to PCOS, and Lalita and Parvati held that menstrual issues resulted from "no proper eating time." Shefali agreed: "They eat late. That causes lots of problems. Acidity increases. It affects everything." Irregular schedules—beyond just eating times—also came in for censure. Office manager Swati, aged 51, spoke of women no longer having a regular routine, and Shabana mentioned late bedtimes along with delayed meals. Leela, the college professor mentioned earlier, emphasized sleep:

> This generation is used to staying up late at night. Even up to two and three am. But they still have to wake up in the morning. Then their night-time sleep is insufficient for them.

Preeti, 33 years old, felt that "PCOD has a lot to do with stress and [a lack of] routine." These observations can be seen to be influenced by indigenous health frameworks that emphasize regularity in bodily cycles and structure in schedules. They implied that there were times which were appropriate not just for eating and sleeping but also for other aspects of day-to-day living and that these time prescriptions were no longer being followed.

The detrimental effects of pollutants and animal hormones were also referenced. Sheetal, for example, cautioned,

> What we take [food] is not good. What reaches us—it is hybrid—we don't get food and grains that are the same quality as before. Even if we want vegetables, they have been grown on the tracks [referring to "gutter farms," near railway tracks where vegetables show the presence of heavy metals]. Added to that, they have been nurtured through fertilizers. So many things are done to increase yield, they are reducing quality.

Manju voiced similar sentiments:

> Food was also, that time [earlier], it was healthier, without this, what do you call it—*milavat* [adulteration]. Food was also very original, organic types. Fertilizers etc., that they put on plants to make them grow? That wasn't there. That time they used to give the food original—now *toh* they are giving all artificial everything. Giving injection, things to give the color and all.

Manju went on to blame pollution as well; she believed that it affected the immune system and, from there, the endocrine system. Lalita, too, mentioned declining food quality, a lack of fresh air, and heavy pollution. Meghna, aged 28, linked pollution to adverse effects on the endocrine system, saying that hormonal imbalances were caused by polluted drinking water and food contaminated with pesticide residues. Lawyer Hemant opined that urban women were exposed to far more pollution than were women in rural areas. Aerospace engineer Prashant put it rather more intriguingly: "There [in villages], bodies don't encounter too many unnatural things."

Another aspect linked to a body out of sync with the natural order was that of biomedicines, particularly hormonal medications. Rahul felt that women were "popping pills—pills to push periods forwards, iPills [emergency contraceptive pills]. It's meddling with their [menstrual] cycles." Shefali's views were similar: "I think [bio]medicines play a vital role in hormonal changes. Taking them too, the [menstrual] cycle changes ... these medicines are really strong medicines." Leela, on the other hand, mentioned hormonal medication but blamed a lack of adherence, rather than the medications as such, for resulting in menstrual issues:

> Some [women] don't get [a period] at all for 2–3 months. It's not just that they haven't got it only once; this is repeatedly. They have to take gynecological treatment.... They don't understand the severity. They take partial treatment—they start and then they leave it in between.

28

Meanwhile, Manju was critical of biomedicines in general, especially anti-biotics, and the tendency to "take pills for every small thing" which "affects the gynec system."

My interlocutors were thus suggesting that by misusing pesticides and fertilizers, humans were disrespecting "natural" temporal rhythms and demanding faster results than they should. The food this produced was degraded, reflecting the immorality of their practices, and this went on to damage the human body. The same applied to biomedicines; by focusing on immediate results, biomedicines meddled with the body's rhythms, and convenience ended up trumping holistic approaches that were more suited to long-term wellness.

Balancing the Traditional and the Modern

The last overarching theme running through my interlocutors' responses related to sociocultural changes and the emergence of new gender norms. These gender norms, they suggested, placed new pressures upon women, especially those of work outside the home and of consumption. Meanwhile, older gender norms, which assigned women sole charge of domestic and household responsibilities, had not been entirely dismantled. Thus, women were expected to juggle new responsibilities alongside their older ones. Interlocutors noted that no real household responsibilities fell upon men, and for women, this meant a double burden of work both inside and outside the home. Interlocutors linked this double burden to stress and, from there, to ill health.

Notably, my interlocutors did not, however, criticize women for their professional and educational ambitions. Their comments were far more nuanced, as they sympathized with women for being unable to escape their domestic duties. For example, Neela, aged 38, stated: "They [women] have the pressure of their job as well as—as a woman, the house responsibilities, generally till now responsibility of the household is still on them, no matter how liberated you are." In Marathi, she called this a *taarvarchi kasrat*, or a tightrope act. Neela added that women were constantly feeling torn between their work outside the home and their family, always carrying a sense of guilt and regret that they were neglecting one or the other. A 29-year-old working mother likewise commented that "Women now do a whole lot more stuff. Then you feel you're not doing justice [to everything] ... it's a constant race with time." Thirty-three-year-old Preeti mentioned the stress of tight deadlines, household and financial issues, and career-related competition. Priyanka, aged 24 and in marketing, commented,

> Stress is increasing. For women who are working there is the work–home balance stress. The number of things to get done are a lot

29

more. Women across the board are worrying more—that is the kind of people we are. Today, no one is insulated from stress. There is a lot more going on.

Neha was clear in her indictment of the gendered nature of household work for this state of affairs, even as she referenced the presence of (female) domestic helpers in middle-class homes. "Work–life balance has dropped a lot," she stated. "Home responsibilities all lie with women. Where have we seen men taking initiative? *Bais* [domestic helpers] also call madam [with queries and for direction], not *saab* [sir]."

Meanwhile, Geeta, the homemaker with grown children, was more equivocal. She attributed much of women's heightened stress levels to their increased expectations of themselves:

Working plus there is the home also. I feel that sometimes they cannot tackle both. There is stress of both these sides.... These days basically the lifestyle has become very stressed out. One thing I feel is that these days, women feel they can do everything. They can do—it is not that they are different from the males of the world, but they themselves have more expectations out of themselves. I feel in that stress really increases a lot.

Another interlocutor pointed to the multiple demands on women and their relationship to changing family structures:

There's financial, family stress, travelling stress ... it has just increased over time. More women are working. There's more inflation. Now we have smaller families, so you have to do everything for yourself—earlier, non-working members used to take care. There are more work pressures on women also.

Lalita, aged 47, thought that even women not working outside the home were having to deal with growing levels of stress. This, she said, was because of "Too much competition, you know, for the kids' educations. They are worked up. I feel people nowadays are too stressed out." Sheetal, also in her 50s, linked stress to a lack of rest, especially during menstruation. "We are getting up and doing everything [as men do]," she said, "but this particular thing [menstruation] is only for ladies." Sudhir, the father of a teenage daughter, spoke of shifts in gender norms, saying that in India,

Society is in transition. You want to follow the norms in terms of lifestyles and all that but culturally, there are still pressures on women. It's a sign of a society in transition ... the percentage of working women in urban areas is much higher, but the women are still solely responsible for everything at home.

Forty-two-year-old Rahul summarized all of these perspectives on changing gender norms when he said,

> Because they [urban women] are juggling family life and work life, their monthly cycles are getting rogered [screwed].... They're not able to get enough rest; there is more strain. You got to lie down in a corner and rest [when you get your period], but today it's no excuse ... there is a lot more strain—emotional, physical, mental. There is a guilt factor. For all relationships, women feel like they are not giving as much as they should.

Taken together, interlocutors' comments call attention to the increased participation of middle-class women in the labor market as well as their lopsided shouldering of household responsibilities and domestic duties. While women pursued their career aspirations and took on professional identities, once married, they nonetheless had to balance these with the conventional marital roles of being good wives, mothers, and daughters-in-law. Despite the respite provided by domestic helpers, middle-class women were still tasked with managing these helpers and supervising their work.

The Nutrition Transition

As described in the earlier chapter, India has experienced vertiginous shifts in the political–economic and social realms since 1991. Economic liberalization has led to economic growth, the emergence of new ways of performing middle classness through consumption, and a shift toward consumer culture. The relaxation of trade tariffs, import regulations, and restrictions on businesses has made previously inaccessible consumer products and services more widely available, and economic growth and social mobility have brought them within the reach of consumers earlier denied such choices. Such shifts toward increasing industrialization, urbanization, and globalization are known to result in a trend toward more obesity-related chronic diseases, and research on India indicates that such a trend is well underway.

Much of this can be attributed to dietary shifts and a decrease in physical activity. In India, women are usually engaged in less physical activity than men thanks to the circumscribing of their movements, and studies have shown that women with domestic help show a higher body mass index than women without (Agrawal 2005). This could be attributable to their higher socioeconomic status—and therefore access to more calorie-dense food and labor-saving devices—or to the availability of domestic help resulting in reduced movement within the home. When it comes to food, while there are urban and rural disparities, by and large, economic growth and higher incomes after 1991 have ushered in the higher consumption of dairy products, fats, oils, and sugar (Griffiths and Bentley 2001; Popkin 2001; Shetty 2002). Consumer data demonstrate that this trend continues.

In the mid-1990s, India was a small importer of vegetable oil, but by 1998, it was the world's leading importer (Hawkes 2006: 5). The demand for edible oil has been steadily growing at a compound annual growth rate of 4.43 per cent from 2001 to 2011 (Nagesh 2012: 191), and there has been a move toward higher consumption of *ghee* (clarified butter) and dairy products (Nagesh 2012; Pingali 2007). The consumption of sugar has also increased, and India exceeds the global per capita average consumption of sugars (Gulati and Misra 2014). Expenditure on sugar was INR 71.7 per household per month in 2007, INR 96 in 2008, and INR 129 in 2010 (approximately USD 1.2, USD 1.6, and USD 2.1, respectively) (Nagesh 2012: 193). Moreover, the consumption of processed, sweetened, and high-fat foods is strongly tied to performances of modernity and notions of prosperity (Wilson 2010).

The consumption of packaged foods such as cheese, butter, jam, biscuits, and noodles has also seen sharp increases (Nagesh 2012; Nichols 2017). This is tied to both the greater availability of these foods and their increased acceptance because of shifts in dietary tastes and new conceptions of what constitutes a meal. Non-Indian foods have increasingly entered Indian diets; pizzas, noodles, pastas, and baked goods are ordered in or eaten when dining out. They are also being cooked in Indian homes—especially urban middle- and upper-class homes—as part of regular family meals. This is not a phenomenon limited to the middle and higher socioeconomic strata alone. In my conversations with slum residents and working-class interlocutors in Mumbai, I regularly heard complaints that their children preferred "Chinese" food—by which they meant "Maggi" (noodles)—or "Pepsi" (used as shorthand for all colas), bread, and sandwiches.[2] Eating out has steadily become much more common for this stratum as well.

At the most basic level, the nutrition transition (Popkin 1993, 2006) framework mentioned earlier helps makes sense of these shifts. The framework suggests that economic development, urbanization, and globalization lead to a predictable shift toward diets that are low in fiber and rich in saturated fats, sugar, and refined foods and toward lifestyles that are low in physical activity. This shift in turn goes on to lead to an increase in obesity-related chronic diseases, such as type II diabetes and heart disease. However, reducing the rise in such obesity-related disorders to the twin axes of diet and physical activity obfuscates more than it reveals. As the health geographer Julie Guthman (2012) has pointed out, the body does not function in such a straightforward, mechanistic manner. The endocrine system mediates the conversion of calories to body fat; there are metabolic pathways to obesity that are not directly related to calorie intake and expenditure.[3] The endocrine system itself is affected by environmental factors such as epigenetic influences[4] (see also Chapter 3) and exposure to EDCs.

Focusing merely on the "calories in, calories out" model, which is implicit in the nutrition transition framework, to explain the rise in obesity-related conditions, including PCOS, in post-liberalization India causes us to miss out on how political–economic shifts following 1991 have led to more varied and nuanced changes in sociocultural determinants of health in the country. Instead of revolving solely around diet and physical activity, public discourses about PCOS referenced a deeper change in interactions between bodies and their environments that cannot be captured by the nutrition transition framework.

"A New Normal"

The nutrition transition model ignores how local conceptions of the body, temporal rhythms, and environmental and sociocultural determinants of health are also transformed through accelerated engagement with globalization and neoliberal work structures. Liberalization was seen by the media samples and my interlocutors to have brought new stressors (especially gendered stressors, which I cover further in Chapter 3) and the disruption of the natural order. Prashant, the aerospace engineer in his late 20s, commented about the stress, hectic schedules, and lack of a sense of wellness that characterized contemporary life: "This is the new normal." I would constantly hear people saying that "people nowadays are too stressed out," or that life was no longer "peaceful." In notable contrast to the nutrition transition framework, interlocutors referenced changing diet patterns through the prism of stress. Irregular or improper meal and sleeping times and "no routine" were typically linked to stress and mentioned as having harmed health and wellbeing. Concerns regarding harmony with the natural order were indexed beyond just temporal aspects. Interlocutors emphasized the moral–ecological decay that led to greed, the abuse of nature (including human bodies, seen to be part of the domain of the natural), and a fixation on quick results. This was reflected in environmental degradation. Such observations were not aimed only at women, women with PCOS, or even individuals. Rather, they formed a criticism of societal shifts. Even as I heard complaints about modern lifestyles, I heard a recognition that opting out of or changing these lifestyles was largely beyond the power of the individual. The implication, rather, was that there had collectively been a change for the worse.

I began this chapter by mentioning how it was common to hear individuals over the age of around 35 bemoan the lack of concern about health on display in the habits of those younger than 35. For people of an older generation, who came of age much before liberalization, the daily patterns of living that were deemed normal by younger individuals were seen as incomprehensible as well as reckless. Comparisons with earlier times, when eating out was infrequent, late nights were uncommon, and the pace of life was slower inevitably followed.

Paying attention to public discourses about PCOS, however, shows how these complaints that are seemingly regarding a shift in generational behavior are really a critique of a shift in generational situations. Fieldwork confirmed that eating out and ordering food in was routine for people under the age of 35 (whom I henceforth refer to as young people). I regularly heard people, even women with PCOS, speak of skipping lunch or having extremely late lunches because of work pressures. Late dinners were the norm, as by the time individuals reached home from work after a long commute, it would be anywhere between 9 and 11 pm. Young people constantly complained of a paucity of time and of busy schedules, which made exercise and the timely eating of wholesome, healthy meals difficult. Long hours were also standard; many regularly worked into the late evening or took work home with them at night and over weekends. Interlocutors would also get phone calls or text messages related to work well after work hours. This was not limited to work. Being online for leisure or social networking late at night and in the morning was also typical. Furthermore, late nights and erratic sleeping habits were routine, and I frequently heard individuals complain of insomnia when they did manage to get to bed early. The use of food drugs such as coffee and tea to stay awake was common.

Although interlocutors spoke of issues such as constipation, insomnia, acidity (as related to delayed or skipped meals), and irregular menstrual cycles as indicators of a less than ideal state of wellness, they also spoke of their inability to make the lifestyle changes required to achieve that ideal state. Eating on time, early dinners, or sleeping early were deemed impractical to their circumstances. As I detail in Chapter 3, women with PCOS too felt that their lifestyles were not conducive to the optimal management of the syndrome, but they found themselves unable to make any real changes.

Late nights and long working hours may not seem comment-worthy to audiences familiar with many European and American contexts. Young people in those contexts tend to socialize intensely, sleep late, eat without much regard for nutrition, and show a general indifference toward carefully managing their health. In India, however, this represents a big shift. For one, Indians tend to live with their families for much longer, and within such multigenerational homes, individual routines used to be tied to household meal and sleep times. Furthermore, as mentioned earlier, indigenous frameworks of health, including those of Ayurveda, prize structure and emphasize regularity in bodily cycles such as those of eating, sleeping, digestion, defecation, and menstruation. That focus on regularity is reflected in popular health culture; bodily cycles are ideally expected to be in tune with daily and seasonal cycles. The prescribed patterns of sleeping a few hours after sundown, waking with sunrise, eating four meals of breakfast, lunch, tea, and dinner, defecating upon waking, and menstruating every 28 days (with even a day or two's delay deemed unwholesome) were implicit in my interlocutors' comments.

Prior to 1991, conforming to such a regular routine—at least to a large extent—was not difficult for members of the middle class. Government sector jobs, which set the tone for white-collar employment and which were the mainstay of the middle class—were secure and seldom required individuals to work late. Fewer consumer goods and services meant fewer demands on the monthly household budget. Avenues for consumption-oriented leisure activities—whether eating out or other late-night entertainment—were similarly circumscribed, even in urban areas, and the distractions of the internet, smartphones, and other communications technologies were absent (Fernandes 2000b, 2006; see also Chapter 1).

The consequences of the "defective modernization" following liberalization have meant that new work structures, consumption activities, and communications technologies routinely disrupt ideal, regular daily rhythms. Notions of a regular schedule and balance with the natural order, although still central to popular conceptions of health and wellness, are nonetheless being abandoned in practice. Meanwhile, widespread pollution from the ecological degradation caused by capitalist overexploitation and the deeper penetration of market forces into agriculture, leading to rampant pesticide and fertilizer use, results in continuous exposure to particulate matter, toxicants, and EDCs. A reliance on processed foods and short-term biomedical fixes further takes its toll on wellness. What interlocutors were indicating, through their observations, was how altogether these experiential aspects of the larger political–economic changes after 1991 have meant that where wellness was once implicitly nurtured by the middle-class way of life, in contemporary times, it required much effort and careful lifestyle management to be achieved. The "new normal" was an unhealthy way of living that then went on to lead to chronic disorders and conditions such as PCOS. Whereas men were not immune, the effects on women were seen to be particularly pronounced (an aspect I deal further with in Chapter 3).

Health Since Economic Liberalization

Commentary about PCOS thus speaks to how the structural changes following economic liberalization have promoted a new way of thinking about the body. Where patterns of daily living for the urban middle class had once been regular, routine, and oriented around the body's rhythms, they were now unshackled from such temporal cycles. The body was no longer treated as vulnerable and in need of shielding from seasonal or environmental pressures. Instead, it was treated as plastic and flexible, and it had become an object to be adapted to the compulsions of work and leisure for maximum utility. Temporal norms regarding the body had also changed. Public discourses about PCOS highlighted issues of time and of the lack of stable rhythms related to eating and sleeping. They also referenced the possible toxic influences of exposures to contaminants such as environmental EDCs (through references to pollution or adulteration) that are lacking in conventional biomedical and public health discourses on the rise of obesity, metabolic syndrome, and related disorders. As I will describe in the next chapter, these discourses nevertheless align with emerging biomedical research on the potential links between changes in metabolic pathways, PCOS, and insulin resistance and meal and sleep times (Jacubowicz et al. 2013; Spiegel et al. 2009), disturbed stress responses (Benson et al. 2009), and EDCs in the environment (Palioura and Diamanti-Kandarakis 2015).

Framing changes in health and the rise in metabolic syndrome-related disorders following globalization in terms of transitions in diet and physical activity patterns results in the issue of problem closure. This means that the definition of obesity-related disorders as caused by energy imbalance frames investigations in certain ways. These framings then preclude alternative possible conceptualizations of these disorders (Guthman 2013). However, engaging with popular ecological frameworks of health and public discourses related to health changes can help reveal alternative conceptualizations. These conceptualizations can help uncover the limitations of conventional biomedical and public health framings. Such engagement has the potential to offer deeper, more nuanced understandings of medical conditions, factors that render specific segments of the population vulnerable to them, and the barriers to their management. This, in turn, can aid the development of more effective interventions to address them.

My interlocutors were connecting the increased incidence and prevalence of chronic conditions such as metabolic syndrome disorders in India to societal stressors—not just to diet and exercise. Health issues were used as vehicles to comment on perceived and experienced problems of contemporary "modern" life. The political–ecological framework underlying these discourses connected health to sociocultural factors (such as changes in gender norms and consumer culture), political–economic shifts (such as the restructuring of the labor market, urbanization, and aspirational marketing), and environmental considerations (pollution resulting from capitalist over-extraction and an overreliance on pesticides and chemical fertilizers as a result of changes in agricultural production). Such commentary points to shifts in patterns of living, ideas of temporality, and interactions between bodies and their environments. These are shifts that go beyond changes merely in dietary intake and physical activity. Moreover, in this framework, the body is part of a larger ecological landscape, connected to a natural order (see also Gold 1998; Nichter 2001). Such reasoning reflects a counter to the medicalization of illness that is characteristic of late modernity. Instead of rooting illness in individual biology, public discourses on PCOS were locating medical conditions in political–economic, social, ecological, temporal, and even moral dimensions. As I show in the next chapter, PCOS can be seen to be the embodied manifestation of the biosocial stresses of the shifts referenced in this metamedical commentary and the toxic locations that result from them. Despite the recognition of these larger structural factors, however, when it comes to the management of PCOS, responsibility for behavior and lifestyle change is still placed upon individual women (see Chapter 4).

Notes

1 Although homeopathy did not originate in India, it is recognized as a nationalized medical system through the Government of India's AYUSH (Ayurveda, Yoga, Unani, Siddha, and Homeopathy) ministry.

2 This is a phenomenon not limited to urban areas; similar observations have been made in rural parts of India too (see, for example, Nichols 2017).

3 To put it in crude terms, the "energy balance" or "calories in, calories out" model focuses on caloric intake as the input, with movement as the output; the difference between these two becomes body weight. This model ignores the role of the process of conversion—metabolic pathways and the endocrine system; that is, a more or less "efficient" process can determine how effectively calories get converted to fat.

4 Epigenetics speaks to the body's ability to be affected by its surroundings and to then pass down such effects across generations; these are not genetic differences ("nature") but rather the different expression of genes, as affected by the environment ("nurture").

3

"HORMONES PLAY HAVOC WITH YOUR BODY"

Toxic Locations and PCOS

Indians are prone to metabolic syndrome disorders such as type II diabetes and PCOS. As mentioned in Chapter 2, they have some of the highest rates of type II diabetes in the world (Wells et al. 2016). On average, they develop diabetes almost ten years earlier than their Euro-American counterparts, and 47 per cent of diabetes diagnoses in India occur before the age of 40 (India State-Level Disease Burden Initiative Diabetes Collaborators 2018; Mohan et al. 2017; Singh, Venkat Narayan, and Eggleston 2019). Similarly, Indians[1] present with coronary heart disease early, and the premature onset of both diabetes and heart disease is linked (Leeder et al. 2004; Prabhakaran et al. 2005; Sosale et al. 2016; Xavier et al. 2008). Emigrant populations of Indians in high-income countries also show a higher susceptibility to diabetes than other ethnic groups. For example, individuals with South Asian ancestry in London, UK, had twice to thrice the type II diabetes risk of their counterparts with Caucasian ancestry. Additionally, their diabetes onset was typically five years earlier and at a lower body mass than their Caucasian counterparts (Tillin et al. 2015). Such disparities remain even after adjustments are made for other risk factors, and the inter-population variation cannot be explained by lifestyle factors alone (Diamond 2011; Enas et al. 2007; Gujral et al. 2013; McKeigue, Shah, and Marmot 1991; Mohan et al. 2007; Ramachandran 2005; Razak et al. 2005).

The onset of disease at lower body mass is worth highlighting: studies have repeatedly shown that Indians display several metabolic disturbances associated with obesity even at BMIs (body mass indices) considered conventionally nonobese (Pomeroy et al. 2019; see also Yajnik and Yudkin 2004). This paradox is also known as the Y–Y paradox—based on the last names, Yajnik and Yudkin, of the two endocrinologists to chronicle this phenomenon—or the paradox of the "thin–fat Indian." The Y–Y paradox draws attention to the fact that Indian bodies are often metabolically obese even when they are morphologically thin (Solomon 2016). That is, these bodies are "fat" in terms of health risks even when they are visually relatively "thin." A few years after the phenomenon of the thin–fat Indian was documented, it was found to be so widespread among the Indian population that it forced a rethinking of the BMI cutoffs for the overweight and

DOI: 10.4324/9781003171423-3

obese categories for this population. These categories were revised downward, from the global cutoff of 25 (for overweight) and 30 (for obesity) to 23 and 27.5 respectively for Indians (Misra et al. 2009).

The exact reasons for this susceptibility are debated. Explanations have ranged from low lean mass, that is, muscle mass, among Indians (indeed, South Asians more generally), possibly caused by hot tropical climates and agricultural uncertainties, to low-protein, largely vegetarian diets and maternal malnutrition. Whether these factors represent a genetic susceptibility—that is, a body rendered vulnerable by its genetic makeup—or epigenetic plasticity—which is the body's ability to be affected by its surroundings and to then pass down those effects through generations—is hotly contested. Explanations of agricultural uncertainty and maternal malnutrition, for example, imply widespread shortages of food and an overall malnourished population. These explanations cast India as a land of scarcity and famine, and they cannot account for realities of privilege and inequality. Despite these debates regarding causality, however, the thin–fat tendency among Indians itself is now well established (Pomeroy et al. 2019; Solomon 2016; Wells et al. 2016).

The paradox of the thin–fat Indian troubles notions of the universal body—a standardized body of black-boxed biological characteristics that shows no distinctive variations across sociocultural, economic, or historical contexts. This conceptualization of the body, which is crucial to clinical trials, has proven indispensable for the biological sciences and to biomedical advances. Nevertheless, it ignores realities of local or socially patterned bodily variations. Although scientists and anthropologists alike had noticed differences across ethnic and community groups, there was a general wariness to acknowledge such difference in case it fed into racist agendas.[2] Margaret Lock (1993), however, proposed the term "local biologies" to sidestep racial essentializing but still counter the universal body, removed from and unaffected by its local contexts and life experiences. The framework of local biologies stresses how social and biological processes are entangled in human biological difference. It stresses biological variation as socially—rather than racially—embedded. That is, this work highlights how sociocultural worlds are reflected in biologies (such that biologies vary as a result of sociocultural experiences) rather than assuming that race exists as a product of biology.[3] In pioneering work on menopause in Japan and North America, Lock found that the symptoms women reported as they approached the end of menstruation varied significantly between these places. Lock linked this not just to culturally patterned differences in diet and physical exertion but also to constructions of the menopausal body, expectations regarding that life stage, and what symptoms were deemed important and noticed. Menopause in Japan was not just conceptually but also experientially different from menopause in North America. Lock's work revealed how the cultural and biological domains are "in a continuous feedback relationship of ongoing exchange, in which both are subject to variation" (Lock and Kaufert 2001: 503). Over time, such a continuous relationship of "biosocial differentiation" (Lock and Nguyen 2010: 90) builds and congeals to reveal itself in local biologies, such as through the thin–fat tendency of Indian bodies.

In the earlier chapter, I described changes in the sociocultural determinants of health that have followed upon the economic liberalization of India. How, then, have these political–economic and political–ecological shifts interacted with the thin–fat Indian metabolic tendency? We know that economic liberalization has brought higher rates of PCOS not just among Indian women but specifically among urban middle-class women in contemporary India. What are the processes of biosocial differentiation that are resulting in urban middle-class Indian women exhibiting much higher rates of PCOS than other women? This chapter revolves around these questions and focuses on the mounting pressures placed on urban middle-class women throughout their life course. It explores how the structural burdens brought by economic liberalization have interacted with a thin–fat local biology to result in toxic locations that compromise women's wellbeing and lead to PCOS.

An Ecosocial Approach

Much medical anthropological work on health disparities or on the cultural production of health focuses on the negative effects of stress and sees it as the means through which social inequalities and precarity result in illness and health issues. However, the term "stress" is typically used loosely, referencing anything from environmental demands to individual or community perceptions of these demands to individual or community ability to respond to them (this is a trend with a fairly long history; see also Kasl 1984). While chronic stress—in the sense of repeated and prolonged activation of the hypothalamic–pituitary–adrenal axis—has been linked to negative psychobiological effects through the possible mediating pathway of oxidative stress,[4] such formulations ignore the possibility that some degree of stress may be beneficial. This notion, that all stress need not be "bad stress," is presented in the concept of "eustress," which posits that manageable (as decided by respondent perceptions) levels of life stress may in fact contribute to psychobiological wellbeing (Ashbacher et al. 2013). Nevertheless, within medical anthropological work, stress is typically treated as an inherent evil to which myriad health issues can be attributed. Moreover, it is relied upon as a black box explanation for health disparities, with no elucidation of how exactly—that is, through what biochemical processes—it might be linked to adverse health outcomes.

In a critique that encompasses but goes beyond this reliance on stress as an explanation for poor health outcomes, the epidemiologist Nancy Krieger (1994, 2001) has pointed out that much of the medical anthropological and medical sociological work on health disparities ignores the pathways and biological mechanisms by which inequality, structural vulnerabilities, or social structures are manifested at the site of the body. Krieger argues that by failing to focus on pathways to pathogenesis, such approaches render biology opaque. They therefore rarely manage to go beyond calls for general socioeconomic justice and cannot point to concrete public health interventions. As a corrective, Krieger proposes an ecosocial perspective. This perspective pays particular attention to the biological pathways implicated in the embodiment of social, historical, and ecological structures. In addition, it is sensitive to the cumulative interactions between differentiated exposures and the susceptibilities that result from various social inequalities.

My lay interlocutors in Chapter 2 blamed stress for the emergence of PCOS as a ubiquitous condition among women in contemporary urban middle-class India. However, if we are to avoid the pitfalls that Krieger highlights, we cannot stop at stress as an explanation. In order to truly investigate the structural forces rendering urban middle-class Indian women disproportionately vulnerable to PCOS and in order to be able recommend interventions to address this vulnerability, we must situate PCOS-affected bodies within their toxic environmental, political–economic, and sociocultural locations and identify the biological mechanisms through which this toxicity becomes embodied. Adopting such an ecosocial approach toward data gathered from observations during fieldwork, the experiences of women with PCOS, and the lay epidemiology detailed in the earlier chapter and placing it in the context of scientific evidence related to the syndrome revealed several pernicious feedback loops. These feedback loops, detailed below, are connected to the development and exacerbation of PCOS. They start at a young age and operate across the life course of urban professional middle-class women.

Early Adolescence and a Hypercompetitive Educational Environment

In India, children begin elementary school, consisting of grades (known in India as standards) one to five at age five, and they start secondary school, consisting of standards six to ten, at age ten. At around age 15, students enter junior college (standards 11 and 12), and then they can go on to do their bachelor's degrees. During standards 10 and 12, students undergo two major school-finishing examinations, known as the board exams, after which they apply for entrance into higher educational institutes as well as into fields of study. Students' performances in these exams determine their ability to enter the educational stream of their choices, especially when it comes to highly sought-after fields such as medicine or engineering. Furthermore, admission to such professional courses also depends upon student performance in an additional set of competitive entrance exams that occur directly after the standard 12 exams.

41

For the middle class in India, education carries enormous significance. It is a core value, and educational accomplishment is esteemed as both a marker of and a pathway to success (Donner 2011). In post-liberalization India in particular, education is crucial for the skilled, globally mobile, and professional jobs that are central features of middle-class aspiration and ambition. Secondary school performance—which, as described earlier, determines higher educational opportunities—is therefore thought to determine lifelong success (or failure). As a result, educational expectations of middle-class students are very high. Among the middle class, the tenth year of schooling, when the first of the board exams occurs, is seen as "the year that can break or make you" (Sancho 2016).

Dwindling government investment in education, rising middle-class purchasing power, post-liberalization middle-class cultural politics, and a push toward privatization have transformed the school sector in India in the last two decades, resulting in far more of the work of education occurring outside, rather than within, the school (Kumar 2020). Schools therefore rely heavily on the social and economic capital of the family when it comes to educating students. For example, schools interview parents prior to granting admissions to their children, and middle-class parents—or rather, mothers—are expected and required to supervise their children's homework and after-school preparation (Donner 2006). Moreover, after-school academic coaching classes ("tuitions"), once meant as a corrective for those students needing extra help with a specific subject, have now become the norm for all school subjects once students enter secondary school. In fact, they are common even as early as the primary school level and have become markers of middle-class identity (e.g., Aljazeera 2009; Ghosh 2009; Sancho 2016). Furthermore, the family is not the only source of the educational expectations and pressures placed upon students. Private schools (where middle-class families send their children) and coaching classes build their reputations on how successfully they shepherd their students through the school-leaving examinations, and as a result, they closely monitor student performance (Sancho 2016).

This intense emphasis on education and academic performance means that children's movement decreases, sometimes quite drastically, as they progress through school and enter the higher standards; by secondary school, they lead largely sedentary lives (see also Swaminathan et al. 2011). Besides attending school, students go to daily tuition classes that extend into the early evening. Even after their school and tuition classes, they must tackle heavy homework loads, practice lessons, and examination preparation. My observations and conversations revealed that the paucity of time in their schedules means that sleep and leisure activities suffer. Students often operate on insufficient sleep and disturbed sleep cycles, as they study late into the night or wake early. Very little time is left for play, especially outdoor play, or sports. The problem is further compounded by the lack of available open spaces in cities. Exercise and physical exertion are not prioritized, as also reflected in the comments from interlocutors in Chapter 2 that in India "There is no exercise culture" or that exercise was not "part of our culture" (see also Wilson 2010). Even though physical training is a part of the school curriculum, few schools have enough space for vigorous sports or physical activity, and the time dedicated to physical training, at best an hour and a half to two hours a week, is often commandeered for other subjects. Observations in Mumbai, corroborated by key interlocutors, also suggested that around puberty, girls' physical activity reduces even more than that of boys, as girls start engaging in less vigorous, more gender-segregated play.

Furthermore, students in India are often highly stressed around the years of crucial exams (Bhasin, Sharma, and Saini 2010; Verma et al. 2002). Studies suggest that, thanks to the middle-class focus on education, students from this socioeconomic stratum suffer even more school-related stress than their upper- and lower-socioeconomic strata counterparts (Deb, Chatterjee, and Walsh 2010). This stress is reinforced by the lack of leisure activities, movement, and other outlets. I heard from interlocutors that parents cut off cable TV subscriptions, curtail their children's socializing, or suspend other forms of their children's leisure during the ninth and tenth standards to prevent "distractions" from study. In addition, young adolescents face high degrees of surveillance during these years, as parents supervise studying and closely oversee schedules; in David Sancho's work on the last years of school in urban India, middle-class adolescents' experience of those years is likened to being under "house arrest" (Sancho 2016: 1). Against this backdrop, I found that eating—culturally central to everyday pleasure and social nurturing (Wilson 2010)—was the only sanctioned source of pleasure. Students seek an outlet in eating, and I noticed that parents would frequently offer calorie-dense sugary treats or fried foods to their children to reward as well as to motivate grueling study routines.

Menarche (the beginning of menstruation) has been variously reported to be around ages 9–15 across India (Acharya, Reddaiah, and Baridalyne 2006; Bagga and Kulkarni 2000; Dambhare, Wagh, and Dudhe 2012; Khadilkar et al. 2006; Khanna and Kapoor 2004; Rokade and Mane 2009). The higher secondary standards of drastically reduced physical activity, inadequate sleep, intense stress, and comfort eating therefore coincide with a key time in the developmental cycle, that of puberty. Typically, the time around menarche is a period of decreased insulin sensitivity. This means that the cells in the body become less responsive to insulin, such that more insulin is needed by cells to use the glucose in the blood. Unchecked, such insulin resistance (reduced insulin sensitivity) usually leads to elevated blood sugar levels and, eventually, diabetes.[5] Insulin resistance, as mentioned in Chapter 1, is also linked to PCOS and other metabolic syndrome disorders. Usually, insulin sensitivity returns to pre-pubertal levels a couple of years after menarche (Goran and Gower 2001). However, weight gain—which is a result of insulin resistance—further decreases insulin sensitivity, as do disturbed sleep cycles and inadequate sleep (Everson et al. 1998; Spiegel et al. 2009).

In the context of a highly sedentary, often sleep-deficient, daily routine that revolves around studying, the reduced insulin sensitivity around menarche combines with reduced movement and insufficient sleep to lead to weight gain, which then furthers decreases insulin sensitivity (Moran et al. 2006). One of my endocrinologist interlocutors summarized these effects by saying, "Fat is an endocrine organ." By this, she meant that fat, once stored in the body, affects the endocrine system through aspects such as sensitivity to insulin; fat loss thereafter stops being a simple matter of increasing energy output through activity or decreasing caloric intake. Furthermore, the period between the ages of 9 and 13 is also a significant period in terms of fat metabolism. Weight gain during this period has been tied to a type of early onset obesity (hyperplastic obesity) that is marked by an increase in the number of adipose (fat) cells[6] rather than an increase in the size of those cells alone (Salans, Cushman, and Weismann 1973). Such obesity is less responsive to physical activity and makes weight loss even more difficult (Björntorp et al. 1977). Overall, then, weight gain during this age contributes to decreased insulin sensitivity, which increases susceptibility to PCOS, which leads to stubborn weight gain, which further adversely affects insulin sensitivity, and so on, in a continuous negative spiral. This is exacerbated by the thin–fat Indian tendency, which makes Indian girls more susceptible to insulin resistance and other metabolic disturbances at lower levels of weight gain. Thus, the particularly vulnerable developmental time around menarche is the very same time that urban middle-class Indian girls' susceptible bodies get buffeted from all sides by multiple, cumulative stressors linked to the development of PCOS.

Adolescence and Delayed Intervention

As described, the time that young adolescents are likely to be experiencing the first symptoms of PCOS is also a time of intense stress. Stress affects the hypothalamic–pituitary–ovarian axis, which can manifest as erratic menstruation that is not necessarily related to PCOS. Furthermore, other symptoms of PCOS, such as acne, are normal features of adolescence. It is therefore easy for the early markers of PCOS to be mistaken for signs of adolescence and overlooked. Many of my interlocutors mentioned the presence of menstrual irregularities early in their lives. However, they told me that when they discussed these irregularities with older female relatives— usually mothers, grandmothers, or aunts—the irregularities were not seen as a matter for concern or action. An interlocutor whose periods had been erratic since the age of 12 told me that, at the time, "People kept telling me, 'it's okay, it's just started, 14/15 *ke baad* [after 14/15] it will normalize'." Another interlocutor, who upon getting her period at age 9 had continued to experience menstrual irregularities until around age 13, was told to give her body "time to settle."

The age of puberty has been decreasing the world over. This is known as the secular trend, and it is also in evidence in and across India (Bagga and Kulkarni 2000; Khadilkar et al. 2006; Khanna and Kapoor 2004; Rokade and Mane 2009). The exact reasons for the secular trend are being debated, with explanations ranging from better nutrition to more everyday exposure to EDCs (Delemarre-van de Waal 2005), but it means that girls in India, especially from the middle and higher socioeconomic strata, get their periods a few years earlier than did their mothers. This results in a generational difference in experiences of menarche. The typical menstrual irregularities associated with menarche ought to normalize within one or two years of beginning menstruation, despite earlier onset of menstruation. Nevertheless, older female relatives, recalling their own experiences of later menarche, perceive these irregularities to be normal into late teenage.

Menstrual abnormalities in PCOS often present early, right around menarche (Sheehan 2004). The perception that these early symptoms of PCOS are regular features of adolescence means that young girls are rarely taken to consult doctors or gynecologists to discuss their irregular periods, leading to delays in diagnosing and managing PCOS. The weight loss that is the first line of management for PCOS is much easier to execute early on. As described earlier, the more the weight gained at a younger age, the harder it is to shed, and the more likely it is to exacerbate PCOS symptoms. In addition, intervention becomes more difficult in the already hectic final school year, when there are little time and attention resources to diligently implement and monitor changes in dietary, sleep, and movement patterns.

Early Adulthood and "Modern" Identities

For urban professional middle-class women, biosocial stressors linked to PCOS continue to accumulate even after adolescence. The new pressures to display "modern" identities described in Chapter 1 and a new emphasis on women's educational and professional attainment (prior to marriage) extend the hypercompetitive educational environment into the early 20s. Having a master's or professional degree is now a middle-class norm, not just for men, but also for women, and young women compete for limited admissions into institutes of higher learning and for good grades within their degree programs (Donner 2011; Sancho 2016). After the years of higher education, the years of urban professional women's early careers are similarly marked by the hectic schedules that, as described in Chapter 2, are characteristic of new work structures of the post-liberalization economy which are built around long hours and competition.

Meanwhile, the lifestyle standards portrayed in the aspirational representations of a globally mobile professional middle class that dominate television, movies, and other media images bring additional financial and bodily pressures of consumption, as individuals and families try to "live up"

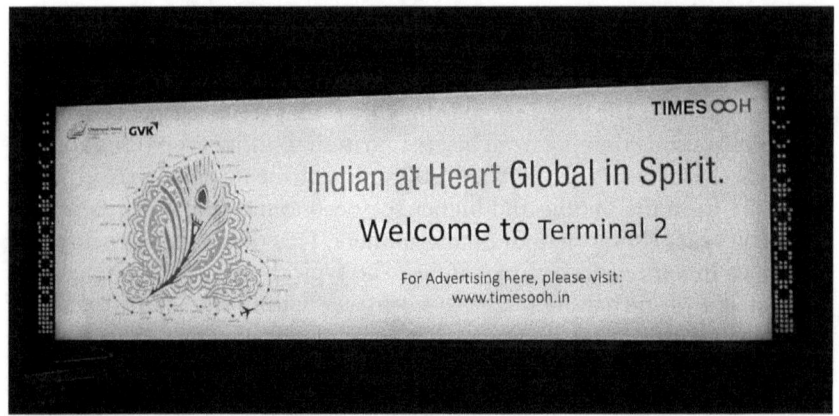

Figure 3.1 Global-yet-Indian as an aspirational ideal advertised at the Chhatrapati Shivaji Maharaj international airport in Mumbai, 2015.

Source: Author

to this consuming and cosmopolitan ideal (see also Chapter 2 and Figure 3.1). Middle-class identities are increasingly tied to the enactment of "modern" identities at the site of the body, and these identities are publicly chronicled through social media for others to see. Interlocutors in their early 20s mentioned lifestyles that revolved around working hard and socializing often. Such lifestyles meant long days, unpredictable meal times, frequent eating out, and late nights. The problem was exacerbated by long urban commutes, which could even go over two hours one way in Mumbai, depending upon traffic. Meanwhile, those unwilling or unable to perform such identities were deemed uncool, unfashionable, or singled out; during my interactions, I regularly heard young women labeled *behenji* (literally sister in Hindi, but with connotations of provinciality and a lack of attractiveness), *paavam* (Tamil word used in the sense of "poor thing"), "aunty" (which holds connotations of being old and frumpy), or as having "no life" by their peers if they didn't frequently party, eat out, or stay up late. These observations were corroborated by Geeta, in her mid-20s, who was trying to eat and sleep better to manage her PCOS: "I'm always the first in the house party to leave, and I'm labelled by my friends for it."

All this makes the interventions required to manage or prevent PCOS extremely difficult to plan and implement (see also Chapter 4). Interlocutors with PCOS spoke often and at length about how challenging it was for them to make diet- or exercise-related changes to their lifestyles given their hectic and unpredictable schedules. Jacqueline, a vivacious 23-year-old with PCOS, described it succinctly: "This is the age [the 20s and 30s] you can't be slowed down, and thinking of health means you have to slow down." Weight gain, sleep deprivation, irregular sleep and meal times, and high levels of stress have all been tied to the development of PCOS, and moving more, early meals, dietary changes, managing stress, and good sleep hygiene are all key to its successful management (Benson et al. 2009; Jacubowicz et al. 2013; Moran et al. 2006; Spiegel et al. 2009). However, for the young women of the urban middle class that I interacted with, long days of work and socializing left little time or energy for regular exercise. Constant eating out and sociocultural imperatives to be seen to be eating—and eating with abandon—made dietary modifications a largely unachievable ideal. In the words of one of my interlocutors, the pressures of "keeping up with the Joneses" in terms of consumption and lifestyles had the inevitable somatic result of "hormones playing havoc with your body."

Marriage, Motherhood, and Balancing the "Modern" with the "Indian"

Ecosocial stressors continue to accumulate even beyond the 20s. Marriage and motherhood are part of the normative biographies of Indian women, and although attitudes to motherhood can be seen to be changing (see Chapter 6), marriage remains a significant life event. As women spend years obtaining higher educational qualifications and working outside the home prior to getting married, the age at marriage among the middle class has been increasing. Nevertheless, once married, women are faced with the double burden of managing their work inside and outside the home. Middle-class women are tasked with performing what scholars have variously called "respectable femininity" (Radhakrishnan 2009), "respectable modernity" (Thapan 2004), or "demure" modernity (Lukose 2009); that is, they are required to balance their performances of modernity, consumerism, and cosmopolitanism with household, familial, and community obligations (Donner 2008).[7] Women are thus expected to be modern/global *and* Indian at the same time. The ability to skillfully navigate these social expectations can affect not only their own social standing but also that of their families (Dickey 2002). In this constant juggling, what constitutes "a good balance" varies according to class, and women of the urban professional middle class have more leeway to engage with the modern (Gilbertson 2014a). However, this leeway also functions as an implicit imperative, and it requires women to move seamlessly between the cultural worlds of work, consumer culture, and the family. They are expected to simultaneously fulfill multiple roles, such as those of a modern consumer, a disciplined professional, a conjugal companion, a dutiful daughter-in-law, and a caring mother. As one interlocutor put it, expectations of women were such that "After coming home [from work] and cooking [for the rest of the family], they still have to get ready and go out to a party if the husband wants to, so he can show off his hot wife."

Careers requiring educational attainment are valued among members of the professional middle-class segment, and although women are expected to prioritize their families over career advancement (Radhakrishnan 2011),

I found that being "just a housewife" was not a desired identity. Interlocutors, even those who had not been working outside the home for many years (usually because they had taken a break after childbirth), referred to themselves by their professions rather than as homemakers. Nevertheless, despite this prizing of professional identities, women were held responsible for the smooth functioning of the household. Even though middle-class women have domestic help, they are still expected to supervise helpers; while they are saved some physical labor, they must shoulder the mental labor of planning, organizing, and managing tasks. For example, recall 27-year-old Neha's description from Chapter 2 that "Home responsibilities all lie with women. Where have we seen men taking initiative? *Bais* [domestic help] also call madam, not *saab* [sir]." In addition, as described earlier, overseeing the children's education—in terms of supervising studies and homework, helping with assignments, and coordinating tuition classes—is the responsibility of mothers; here again, the time commitment and mental labor of planning, organizing, and supporting learning are placed upon women. Unlike men, women are also expected to shoulder the emotional labor of caring for and catering to the needs of the larger family, whether natal relatives or affinal ones.

For my interlocutors, all of this further contributed to inadequate sleep and swamped schedules with little time, energy, or mental space for the planning and implementation of dietary changes, sleep regularization, or exercise regimens that could help manage PCOS. Moreover, I found that lifestyle interventions—particularly dietary ones—were complicated to implement as they required the participation and support of the entire household rather than the participation of just the individual woman. Commenting on these challenges, one interlocutor noted,

> Who is deciding the diet? They [the household] order a chicken biryani—somebody has to finish it. She [the woman] is finishing leftovers, eating the wrong food, and catering to so many people. She can't cook a healthy meal. If she cooks a salad, the mother-in-law says "You are starving my son!"

Throughout all these life stages, as a result of urban living, women are simultaneously exposed to an assortment of EDCs through their daily routines and in their environments and to constant sensory stimuli in the form of city noises, billboards, and bright lighting. These further disrupt endocrine systems and circadian (body clock) rhythms, exacerbating hormonal issues even more (e.g., Kandaraki et al. 2010; Kang et al. 2015). Meanwhile, the configurations of urban space have been changing. Major construction projects revolve around roadworks or residential and commercial real estate and parking, reducing green cover and open space. As more cars find themselves onto Indian roads, roads get choked with traffic, and as public land, such as that on sidewalks, is claimed for illegal constructions or for slum areas inhabited by a continuous stream of new migrants to cities, there are fewer areas left for casual play or everyday walking, reducing opportunities for movement. Together, all these ecosocial factors synergize to create a perfect storm that helps overdetermine PCOS. They also magnify the long-term health risks brought by PCOS, such as the risk of developing type II diabetes. The cumulative effect of these exposures worsens PCOS outcomes.

Structural Burdens and Local Biologies

In pointing to these ecosocial stressors among urban middle-class women, I am by no means suggesting that they face greater pressures than women of other socioeconomic strata, particularly women who may be of the less-than-middle classes. Neither do I wish to imply that these stressors are unique to women in India as opposed to elsewhere. What I do argue, however, is that the unique combination of the new pressures among women in this stratum, combined with their local biology, has contributed to making urban professional middle-class women India particularly vulnerable to PCOS, and it has led to a rise in PCOS cases among this class segment. These women are caught in a toxic location—as a result of their local biology, political–economic context, and urban geography—that is linked to the development of PCOS.

The focus on education among the middle class and the examination pressures among middle-class students in India are not new. What is noteworthy, though, is the degree of competition, which has been progressively growing, experienced by students since the restructuring of the schooling sector in the 1980s and 1990s. Furthermore, new expectations on women to do well in the last couple of decades—whether for success on the job or the marriage market (see Chapter 1)—have made competition even fiercer, with boys and girls now competing for opportunities which were once largely the preserve of boys. As mentioned in Chapter 2, since liberalization, the rhythms of daily living—whether of waking, eating, or sleeping—have been transformed among the urban middle class as a result of the compulsions of work and consumption-oriented leisure activities. Similarly, women have always shouldered responsibility for the household and work within the home in India, but earlier, middle-class women were largely discouraged from working outside the home upon getting married. Middle-class women are now recruited to be prolific consumers *and* producers within the post-liberalization political–economic landscape. The financial pressures of middle-class consumption in the post-liberalization era, injunctions to be "global-yet-Indian," and class identities built around the educational and professional status of women have led to a growing double burden on urban professional middle-class women of work inside and outside the home.

Pressures related to this double burden as well as those of performing consumer cosmopolitanism are, of course, not unique to post-liberalization

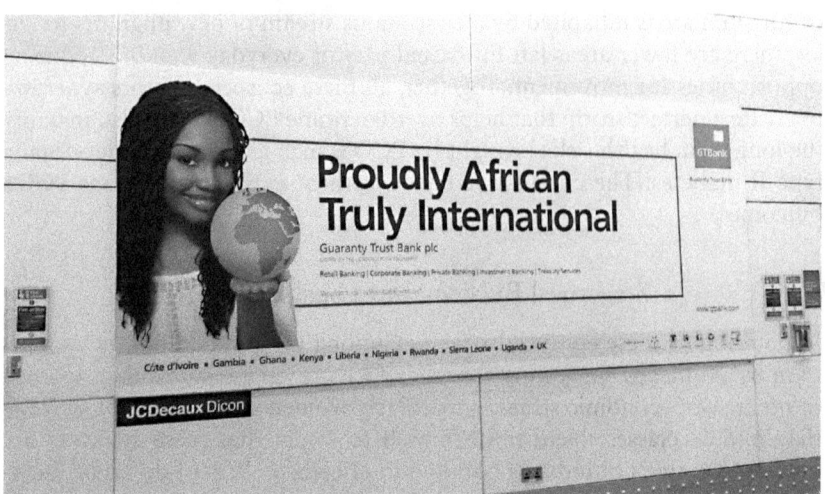

Figure 3.2 Local-yet-global identities advertised outside India; photo taken at Heathrow airport, 2016.

Source: Author

India. However, the combination of the interaction between these new stressors and a specific local biology—that of the thin–fat Indian tendency that predisposes bodies to metabolic disorders—*is* unique to India. Together, they result in urban middle-class women in India being more prone to developing PCOS than middle-class Indian women of previous generations as well as women in other geographical, sociocultural, and local biological contexts.

In 2016, as I transited Heathrow airport in London, a sign featuring an advertisement for a bank proclaimed, "Proudly African Truly International" (Figure 3.2). The sign suggested to me that the "global-yet-local" identity was not prized in India alone. How does the pursuit of this identity affect the health of women in other countries and regions? PCOS has been tied to middle-class lifestyles not just in India but also in the Middle East and elsewhere (Inhorn 2015). Will these regions, which are also experiencing shifts in aspiration and pressures to exhibit "modern" or "global" lifestyles, witness similar increases in PCOS? How will their local biologies affect PCOS outcomes? What do PCOS outcomes look like in other countries with notoriously grueling examination systems, such as in China, South Korea, or Singapore? These questions, while beyond the scope of this book, would be worth exploring in order to place the experiences of PCOS among Indian women in a global context.

What about the less-than-middle classes in urban India? More epidemiological research is needed into how the pressures of modern living relate to PCOS, broken down by socioeconomic strata. Women from the less-than-middle classes face their own array of chronic biosocial stressors—from poverty and precarity to higher degrees of intimate partner violence and struggles for food and sleep. In Euro-America, these are the classes where type II diabetes, heart disease, and other metabolic syndrome disorders tend to be most prevalent (Connolly et al. 2000; Paeratakul et al. 2002; Xu et al. 2017). In India, at the time of writing this, metabolic syndrome disorders are still largely diseases associated with the more affluent classes. That, though, may be changing. Studies from India suggest that the urban poor are beginning to exhibit higher rates of obesity, coronary heart disease, and type II diabetes, although not yet at the same levels as the middle and higher socioeconomic strata (Gupta et al. 2003; Misra et al. 2001). My own experience of volunteering at free medical camps in urban slums in Mumbai suggests that PCOS may not be too far behind—the volunteer doctors and I observed many of the typical clinical features of PCOS, such as overweight or cystic acne, and heard complaints regarding delayed or absent menstrual cycles. Whether the experiences of PCOS for women within these classes will be similar to those of women from the urban professional middle class and whether many of the ecosocial factors implicated in PCOS in women among this middle-class segment will be replicated or even heightened in lower or rural socioeconomic strata remain to be seen.

Toxic Locations

In the earlier chapters, I described the political–economic shifts that followed the liberalizing of the Indian economy and how these shifts have affected sociocultural determinants of health. By chronicling people's opinions on emerging health conditions such as PCOS, I pointed to a new relationship between the body and its environment among the urban professional middle class in post-liberalization India. In this chapter, I have focused on the specifics of how those political–economic shifts and this new relationship between the body and its environment are implicated in the development of PCOS and the worsening of PCOS outcomes. My aim in this chapter has been to stay focused on the biological pathways through which sociocultural contexts and structural burdens become embodied, moving beyond a reliance on and reification of the broad, black-boxed category of stress alone.

Contemporary urban middle-class living places unique structural burdens on Indian women, which, when they interact with the thin–fat local biology, are implicated in rising rates of PCOS among this class. These structural burdens are linked to the pressures of aspiration and globalization, especially the pressures of embodying "modern-yet-Indian" identities. Although urban middle-class women (especially women of the professional middle-class segment) enjoy a position of privilege in India, they are nevertheless situated in a toxic location, at the interface of multiple, interacting, and cumulative ecosocial factors linked to the health pressures of globalization and economic liberalization. Indeed, these ecosocial factors—and their biological manifestations—can in fact be viewed to result from their relative privilege and the gains made from economic liberalization.

To date, research on health disparities and their links to structural and socioeconomic factors has tended to focus on socially or economically marginalized populations (e.g., Baer 1996; Farmer 1999; Holmes 2011; Kim et al. 2000; Navarro 2002; Quesada, Hart, and Bourgois 2011; Singer and Clair 2003; Weaver and Mendenhall 2014). Such studies are, of course, crucial to highlighting the multifaceted and complex health effects of socioeconomic inequalities and to imagining and working toward a more just world. However, ignoring the health outcomes that can result from non-marginalized toxic locations risks eliding a true picture of the human manufacture of risks and the costs to wellbeing attendant upon our contemporary globalized capitalist–industrial order as it becomes even more deeply entrenched, especially in regions of the Global South. Recognizing the toxic location that urban professional middle-class women in India are situated in is one step toward that goal. In the next chapter, I examine how women from the urban professional middle-class segment engage with healthcare practitioners and medical technology to help them navigate the health consequences of that location.

Notes

1 Although this tendency is also seen in other South Asians, I shall restrict myself to Indians here.
2 The acknowledgment of such difference could have been used to support notions of the biological roots of racial difference. Research has, however, consistently shown that race cannot be clearly biologically delineated, that it is an inadequate explanation for human variation, and that there tends to be much more variation within races than between races (Goodman 2000).
3 Nevertheless, such work recognizes that race, as a sociocultural construct, has effects—in terms of other health-related variables such as experiences of discrimination, inequality, and privilege—that can affect health outcomes and result in patterned biological disparities.
4 One way of thinking of the relationship between oxidative stress and ill health is in terms of damage to cells.
5 Insulin resistance is therefore often referred to as pre-diabetes.
6 Hyperplastic obesity differs from hypertrophic obesity, which is an obesity marked by an increase in the size—rather than number—of adipose cells. Hypertrophic obesity tends to have a later age of onset than hyperplastic obesity.
7 I do not mean here to give the impression that discourses regarding the balancing of a global "modernity" with a national "tradition" in the performance of femininity are a recent phenomenon; the relationship between the nation and the appropriate middle-class female subject goes far beyond the neoliberal economic reforms that gained traction in the 1990s and can trace its roots to the burgeoning nationalist movement of the colonial period. What is novel—and pertinent to the present study—is the degree to which women are expected to engage with the "modern" and the kinds of bodily performances that this entails.

4

"HEALTH IS NO MORE
A PRIORITY"

PCOS and Clinical Encounters

The early 19th century saw a shift in Britain's colonial rule of India, such that it came to be increasingly marked by the logics of a civilizing mission. The legitimacy and cultural authority provided by science was central to this endeavor; the British colonial power framed itself as superior because of its access to science and reason. Indigenous Indian forms of science and medicine were devalued as baseless, and India's otherness from Britain was represented in terms of disease and dirt. Science and medicine were harnessed to position the colonizer as a benevolent pastoral force, while the colonized Indians were treated as superstitious, irrational subjects in need of educating. As a result of this framing, science and medicine became key to India's anti-colonial nationalist project. The Western-educated elite in India enthusiastically took to science, and Indian scientists began to selectively incorporate elements from Indian—usually Hindu—"tradition" to construct an Indian modernity. In a bid to deny that a scientific temperament was alien and unsuited to the country, the Indian nationalist project also began to mine tradition to construct a narrative of a golden scientific past. Ayurveda, as an indigenous system of medicine, was championed by the nationalist project as an example of such a typically Indian science (Arnold 2000; Prakash 1999). Similarly, homeopathy—although not indigenous to India—was embraced for the challenge it represented to the hegemony of colonial medicine (Prakash 1999). Both these systems of medicine remain popular to date.

This colonial history is reflected in the Indian state's recognition of not just biomedicine but also homeopathy and the indigenous medical systems of Ayurveda, Siddha,[1] and Unani Tibb.[2] Medical pluralism is entrenched in popular health culture, and these diverse systems of medicine are not viewed as being exclusive of or contradictory to each other. In medical and popular practice, shifts from one system to another or the concurrent use of two or more systems is not unusual. Practitioners often prescribe medications and therapy from two or more systems. A type of "masala medicine," in which therapeutic modality is suited to the individual patient's preferences, finances, and needs, is common (Nichter 1980).

DOI: 10.4324/9781003171423-4

Among the lower socioeconomic strata, shifts between systems of medicine tend to be pragmatic rather than based on the nature of disease (Nichter 1996). Among the professional middle-class segment, however, I found that there seemed to be a clear division of use between biomedicine (commonly referred to as allopathy) and indigenous systems of healthcare. Allopathy was the medicine of choice for acute or urgent medical conditions or for quick relief from symptoms that were felt to hamper daily functioning. Although prized for its ability to offer quick relief, however, allopathy was viewed as being symptomatic and atomistic in approach. As mentioned in Chapter 2, anxieties about the "side effects" of allopathic treatments, especially medications, and their consequences on the body and on future wellness were common. For chronic conditions or issues related to a feeling of general wellbeing, professional middle-class interlocutors therefore drew upon homeopathy and, to a lesser degree, Ayurveda; they were thought to take holistic approaches to health and therefore to be more suited to optimizing wellness. These medical systems, while seen as less effective in the case of emergencies or acute problems, were considered particularly suited to complaints that allopathy could not recognize or adequately address. However, I found that even though Ayurveda was respected in theory, fears generated by reports about heavy metals and adulterants in unregulated Ayurvedic medicines (see, for example, Saper et al. 2008) affected its popularity among the professional middle-class segment. Interlocutors therefore largely preferred standardized food supplements touted as Ayurvedic or herbal instead.[3] Nonetheless, it was typical among this class segment to engage with multiple therapies simultaneously, especially biomedicine, homeopathy, folk medicine (i.e., kitchen remedies), and supplements/herbal medicines sold as Ayurvedic. I did not hear from any of my participants or interlocutors about the use of Unani Tibb or Siddha.

PCOS, as a chronic condition with visible symptoms, is considered suitable for allopathic treatment as well as for treatment by homeopathy and Ayurveda. Furthermore, given the diversity in physical—and often culturally unattractive—symptoms that result from PCOS, such as irregular menstruation, subfertility, insulin resistance, weight gain, cystic acne, hirsutism, scalp hair loss, and acanthosis nigricans, women seek contact with a variety of medical and paramedical professionals to diagnose and manage the condition. In this chapter, I focus on this patient–practitioner contact.

Diagnostic Itineraries

PCOS symptoms fall into three main clusters: skin and hair concerns, menstrual and fertility concerns, and weight and insulin resistance concerns. As a result, women with PCOS typically visit dermatologists, gynecologists, and endocrinologists, depending upon their symptoms. Besides this, they also consult dietitians or nutritionists for help with losing weight and homeopaths and Ayurvedic practitioners (*vaidya*) for overall wellness.

My interviews with these practitioners and interactions with women with PCOS revealed that the diagnosis and management of PCOS tended to follow a few common trajectories, depending upon symptoms and life stages.

Dermatologists

As described in the earlier chapter, early diagnosis, that is, diagnosis of PCOS during adolescence, is rare. Among my interlocutors with PCOS, the condition had typically been identified only once women were in their 20s. Many of the women with PCOS whom I spoke to and interacted with had visited dermatologists for their symptoms before receiving their diagnosis; the dermatologists were instrumental in their condition being identified. The most common complaint was persistent and severe acne, followed by hirsutism, especially in terms of hair on the upper lip and chin. My dermatologist interlocutors explained that women with PCOS present with acne that is predominantly cystic or inflammatory, which tends to be concentrated near the lower cheeks and jawline. Such cystic acne is stubborn and resistant to typical first-line therapies such as topical antibiotics, exfoliants, and retinoids. Acne associated with (unmanaged) PCOS also gets exacerbated, rather than mitigated, with age, and it may be adult-onset acne that appears in the mid- to early 20s, after—rather than during—puberty and adolescence. Most of the dermatologists that I spoke to mentioned that the presence of such stubborn adult acne, combined with hirsutism, overweight, or menstrual irregularities, led them to suspect PCOS. To confirm this diagnosis, they would recommend a sonography. If the sonography showed the presence of polycystic ovaries, women were diagnosed as having PCOS and referred on to gynecologists or endocrinologists.

However, not all women with PCOS who visited dermatologists presented with menstrual irregularities. One dermatologist remarked that up to 70 per cent of patients with PCOS who visited her did not demonstrate menstrual issues. Another dermatologist, Dr. Desai, explained:

> They are not frank [clinically evident] PCODs. They are just on the verge of say, having menstrual—most of these are also not having frank menstrual irregularities, but when probed—they never say they have irregularities—but when probed, they say, yeah, last month, or one or two months, they've had a little irregularity, in the sense the period is still not come or was delayed last month. That is the reason that they are not frank, but the skin features are there. I feel that the skin features precede frank PCOD.

Thus, in practice, skin complaints (along with overweight) were some of the earliest symptoms, and dermatologists were picking up on borderline PCOS or identifying the condition before it began to manifest in gynecological aspects.

The presence of overweight or obesity is significant here. Weight gain is a major clinical marker through which medical practitioners suspect PCOS. As I detail later in this chapter, this has implications for women who do not present with weight gain or high BMIs. All the five dermatologists that I interviewed were aware of and acknowledged the "lean PCOS" phenotype (see Chapter 1), in which PCOS does not manifest as evident overweight or obesity, but three felt that women with such a phenotype were very rare. One even commented about lean PCOS, "It is scarce. I'll have to think; it is that less.... If they are not obese, they are at least well built. On the upper side of normal." Observation and interviews revealed, however, that in cases where women were not overweight, if stubborn adult acne could not be resolved within a few months of treatment, dermatologists recommended diagnostic tests to rule out PCOS. Overall, dermatologists were one of the first medical practitioners *en route* to a PCOS diagnosis, especially for women for whom menstrual irregularities were not entrenched.

I was told by dermatologists that the majority of their patients with PCOS had come to them in their 20s and early 30s, although there were rare instances of girls coming to them in their teens or of women in their 40s consulting them. Teenagers were focused on combating acne and acne scars, or, in some cases, dealing with severe hirsutism. More often, though, women would consult dermatologists either prior to beginning a search for grooms through arranged marriage channels or prior to the wedding. Dr. Pillai explained:

> Looking for grooms, hirsutism is a major issue and these girls [with hirsutism] are quite emotionally disturbed. There are young girls who are in their late teens or early 20s who get teased by boys in school, college, "Hey you know you're getting a mustache," and like this and all that.... But there is a spurt in the number of, in the timing of the girls, and boys also [with acne, who consulted her], because they are going to start looking for spouses in the next couple of months. Mothers who refused to take the girls to the doctor for acne would themselves bring the girl because after one month, you know, somebody is gonna come [to visit her as a prospective bride].

Dr. Fernandes had similar observations:

> Many a times the parents bring the daughters along cause when they've reached a marriageable age, and they are looking for, you know, a suitable partner, then they want to, you know, the girl has to look presentable. So they want a clear skin. So generally before they start the whole process.... Some of them are rejected [for skin or hair problems]. Among certain communities, it is like, you know,

the girl doesn't look so very—presentable, then the amount of dowry that the father has to shell out is quite a bit. So it is taxing to the parents.

The other theme when it came to life stage and consultations from patients with PCOS was of women who were working in marketing or the hospitality industries seeking help in their 20s and early 30s. Dr. Pillai elaborated:

There is a category of girls particularly who work in the hospitality industry; for them, it is for themselves as well as for the job. Little acne also is not tolerated in cabin crew and hotel front office staff. Yeah, so then...there are "grooming officers." You've not heard of this? Airlines have grooming officers; they are officers at a certain job anyway, but they are in charge of grooming, and they tell these girls, they point out, you know, "take care of this." Beyond a certain point, if they don't take care, they are "grounded," if they are at an airline. They are grounded.

Dr. Fernandes seconded this observation, stating, "I've had airhostesses who have been grounded because of pimples or you know whatever." Women with PCOS visited dermatologists to address skin and hirsutism issues, and their motives for such visits included instrumental reasons, such as for careers or in order to improve their prospects for an arranged marriage, as well as more intrinsic motivations, such as wanting to look presentable for their own self-esteem (I examine this further in Chapter 6).

Gynecologists

Gynecologists were the other medical practitioners to diagnose PCOS. Women would approach gynecologists for menstrual issues, such as irregular, delayed, or absent periods, and for fertility issues related to delays in conception. Although women would sometimes visit gynecologists after having already gotten a sonography (recommended by dermatologists or, as I found out, sometimes by family members who were doctors),[4] in many cases, gynecologists would be the ones to recommend diagnostic tests and a sonography to diagnose PCOS. A pelvic sonography (rather than a transvaginal one, which was considered inappropriate for unmarried women) was the most commonly recommended diagnostic investigation, but some gynecologists said they would suggest supplementary hormonal assays to rule out thyroid dysfunction and to check testosterone levels. The type of testing varied—some gynecologists told me that they recommended fewer tests for women of the lower socioeconomic strata, who were likely to find the costs of testing prohibitive. Notably, most of my interlocutors with PCOS did not mention having had tests other than an ultrasound in order to get the PCOS diagnosis; diagnostic investigations recommended by gynecologists seemed to be more common once women consulted these practitioners in order to conceive. My gynecologist interlocutors told me that they relied mostly on the presence of clinical features, such as delayed or absent menstrual cycles, obesity, acne, and hirsutism, to identify PCOS. Confirmation from an ultrasound would then lead them to deliver a PCOS diagnosis.

Women with PCOS usually visited gynecologists at two life stages: (1) in their early 20s, often as they started the process of searching for grooms though arranged marriage channels or (2) in their late 20s and early 30s, after a couple of years of unsuccessfully trying to conceive. An incident from my fieldwork may prove illustrative here: as I sat in gynecologist Dr. Joshi's office to interview her, a woman knocked. Upon being told to enter, she asked Dr. Joshi if her daughter would be okay, following that with, "Doctor, she will be able to conceive, no?" Dr. Joshi asked if the daughter was married. "No, doctor, we are looking for boys," was the reply. Dr. Joshi went on to assuage the mother's fears by saying:

> These days with treatments there is no reason for anybody not to have a biological child. And sometimes even if you have no problems you will not be able to have a child. All this is God's doing. Don't worry about this. Nothing to worry about.

After the mother left, Dr. Joshi explained—the woman's 22-year-old daughter had just been diagnosed with PCOS. Such incidents, she added, were not unique. Other gynecologists reiterated this observation; one gynecologist said that he had parents bring daughters of "marriageable age with irregular cycles to be healthy before everything [wedding-wise] is done." Others spoke of this being much more common among certain communities (e.g., Marwadis and Gujaratis, considered to be "business communities" that were more conservative in terms of gender norms) or among the less-than-middle classes. Besides this, gynecologists also spoke of women in their early 20s seeking help for menstrual irregularities because such irregularities were viewed as a general wellness issue (see Chapter 2) regardless of matrimonial preparations. Whereas the first life stage at which women became concerned about menstrual issues was the one around the time of marriage, the second revolved around motherhood. Married women would visit gynecologists if they had not become pregnant after two to three years of trying to conceive, seeking to address possible subfertility and reproductive issues.

Therapeutic Itineraries

Once women were diagnosed, the work of management commenced. This involved gynecologists but also endocrinologists, homeopaths, *vaidya*, dietitians/nutritionists, and, to a lesser degree, dermatologists. The work of management also involved three therapeutic modes: (1) medication and medical technology, (2) dietary strategies, and (3) other lifestyle interventions. Although these lines are, in theory, supposed to overlap, as I detail below, more often than not, medication became the primary therapeutic mode.

Dermatologists

Typically, dermatologists referred patients with a PCOS diagnosis to other medical practitioners—usually gynecologists or endocrinologists—for overall management. As a result, they largely dealt with only the skin- or hair-related aspects of PCOS and did not have to proffer lifestyle advice or advice about interventions to reduce PCOS patients' risks of diabetes and insulin resistance. Nevertheless, three dermatologists mentioned that they recommended general dietary changes (cutting down refined carbohydrates), increased movement, and stress management techniques, such as yoga, breathing exercises, and meditation. Therapy, however, mostly focused on medications, such as topical treatments for acne and hair loss, and the use of medical technology, such as laser hair removal for hirsutism.

Gynecologists

Gynecologists were the most commonly consulted medical practitioners for PCOS, and management varied depending upon life stage. For unmarried women, gynecologists recommended limited cycles of oral contraceptives. Women were advised to take oral contraceptive pills for three to six menstrual cycles to stabilize their periods. After this, they were advised to stop the medication and check if their menstrual irregularities had been addressed. Gynecologists usually discouraged the prolonged use of oral contraceptives, as they were seen as harmful in the long term not just by the doctors themselves but also by patients or patient's relatives. As a therapy, oral contraceptives were not aimed at menstrual issues alone. They also helped mitigate acne issues, although gynecologists would sometimes refer women to dermatologists for other topical treatments for skin and hair concerns. Some of the gynecologists I spoke to would also routinely prescribe insulin sensitizers, which increase insulin sensitivity, to their overweight or obese patients, sometimes even without a glucose tolerance test (to test for insulin sensitivity) or other investigations. The experiences of my interlocutors with PCOS suggest that such prescriptions were very normal. Women could not, however, articulate the relationship between insulin resistance, weight gain, diabetes risk, and menstrual issues. That is, my conversations with women with PCOS suggested that these links were either not explained to them by their gynecologists or not explained in a manner that encouraged recall.

For married women, some gynecologists would advise early pregnancies—women were encouraged to have children before their fertility underwent further age-related declines. Such advice was also mentioned by my interlocutors with PCOS; they pointed to it as a source of anxiety when they were early into their marriages and did not feel ready for parenthood but had not decided to be childless either (see Chapter 5). For couples that were not immediately planning pregnancies, gynecologists would recommend limited cycles of hormonal contraceptives, just as they did for unmarried women.[5] In the case of patients who had been unsuccessfully trying to conceive, those women were prescribed ovulation inducers. If the ovulation inducers did not result in a successful pregnancy, couples would be advised to consult fertility specialists or to consider in vitro fertilization (IVF) and other assisted reproductive technologies. Some gynecologists also referred women to endocrinologists if there was evidence of insulin resistance—though most gynecologists treated this themselves by prescribing insulin sensitizers—or thyroid dysfunction.

In terms of dietary changes or other lifestyle interventions, gynecologists focused their advice on overweight or obese patients, and it revolved around losing weight. The degree of sensitivity with which the topic was broached and the level of detail provided varied across gynecologists. Some merely mentioned the need for weight loss or recommended that women sought advice from nutritionists, whereas others explained the syndrome's links to type II diabetes and the importance of cutting down on refined carbohydrates and of getting more exercise. None of the gynecologists I interviewed mentioned advising PCOS patients regarding changes to their lifestyles in terms of stress management or getting more—and more regular—sleep; diet was the primary target of their lifestyle-based advice.

Endocrinologists

Endocrinologists were the other biomedical practitioners consulted in relation to the overall management of PCOS. Women visited endocrinologists after referrals by dermatologists, gynecologists, or relatives who were doctors. By the time women visited endocrinologists, they would usually have a PCOS diagnosis and ultrasound report already in hand. The endocrinologists would therefore be "secondary consults." In some cases, women would seek out endocrinologists themselves after receiving an ultrasound report showing polycystic ovaries and being told by the radiologist that PCOS is a hormonal disorder.

Unlike gynecologists, who treat PCOS as largely a reproductive and menstrual condition, endocrinologists view it as an endocrine system disorder. For them, a PCOS diagnosis is a diagnosis of exclusion. This means that the diagnosis requires not just the presence of symptoms and clinical features, but also the elimination of other potential explanations for those features. Endocrinologists in general asked women to conduct a hormonal profile before commencing treatment. Diagnostic testing was therefore heaviest when consulting endocrinologists, as they recommended hormonal assays (e.g., for androgen levels), glucose tolerance tests to test for insulin resistance, and tests to rule out complications or other hormonal conditions that can cause symptoms similar to PCOS (thyroid dysfunction, Cushing's disease, congenital adrenal hyperplasia, hyperprolactinemia, etc.).

Women with PCOS would come to endocrinologists at various life stages and with varied symptoms, whether hirsutism, acanthosis nigricans, insulin resistance, obesity, high cholesterol, thyroid dysfunction along with PCOS, or fertility issues; this last was especially true in the case of reproductive endocrinologists. Standard lines of treatment included medication such as hormonal contraceptives to regularize periods and stabilize hormonal fluctuations, anti-androgens, or insulin sensitizers. In the case of other metabolic conditions or hormonal issues (such as thyroid dysfunction or high cholesterol) along with PCOS, endocrinologists recommended medication to target these comorbidities. Women with subfertility issues were sometimes prescribed ovulation inducers. Endocrinologists were the most likely to stress the links between PCOS and other metabolic conditions, and they routinely recommended dietary interventions (most advised patients to seek help from clinical nutritionists) and lifestyle changes in terms of increased exercise, and, occasionally, stress management; sleep was not mentioned.

Nutritionists and Dietitians

During fieldwork, I found that the terms *nutritionist* and *dietitian* were used interchangeably, even though there was a wide variation in the qualifications of these practitioners, from professional degrees to short certificate courses; individuals can practice as dietitians even with a post-graduate diploma. Some hospitals or endocrinology practices had clinical nutritionists who specialized in the dietary management of medical conditions (henceforth referred to as clinical nutritionists) attached to them. However, dietitians or nutritionists as such did not always have experience with dietetics for medical management (henceforth referred to as dietitians).

For dietitians, weight loss, rather than nutritional management, was the primary focus. Interviews revealed that most dietitians had been trained under a system that viewed all fats as the enemy; most were not familiar with developments in nutrition science that had brought increased attention to glycemic indexes and that implicated carbohydrates, especially simple or refined and highly processed carbohydrates (sugar, high fructose corn syrup, white bread, white rice, flour, etc.), in obesity and metabolic disorders. Women with PCOS, too, visited dietitians primarily in order to lose weight, whether after unsuccessfully attempting to do so on their own or upon the advice of their doctors. Generally, dietitians' clientele comprised (1) teenagers and college-aged young women worried about their weight, (2) young women around the age where they began seeking arranged marriage alliances, (3) women in their late 20s and early 30s advised by endocrinologists or gynecologists to lose weight to aid conception, or (4) older women who had been diagnosed with health complications such as insulin resistance (pre-diabetes) or diabetes and who had therefore been advised to lose weight. None of my slim interlocutors with PCOS had visited dietitians or clinical nutritionists, and none of the dietitians I interviewed had been consulted by women with PCOS who were not overweight or obese.

Of the five dietitians/nutritionists I interviewed, only two knew of dietary specifications for PCOS. The dietary management of PCOS typically involves diets that are low in carbohydrates, especially sugar and simple carbohydrates (which are carbohydrates that are easily digested), and that are built around low glycemic index[6] foods, higher fiber, and adequate levels of protein. One of the two interlocutors who mentioned these specifications was a clinical nutritionist. Of the remaining three, two had only come to know about PCOS as a result of clients with the syndrome visiting them; their advice was to reduce eating out, to eat more soups and salads, and to move to low-fat diets. They especially recommended that women with PCOS reduce their use of oil or *ghee* (clarified butter) when cooking and that they minimize the volume of fried foods in their meals. Most dietitians recommended daily walks to increase physical activity but did not recommend much exercise beyond that. Indeed, one dietitian actively *discouraged* her clients from moderate to heavy exercise. She told me that she believed that once individuals started exercising, they would need to constantly increase their levels of physical activity in order to keep their weight stable; that is, she believed that the body would become habituated to exercise, such that it would require escalating physical activity to maintain the same weight.

Homeopaths

As a result of the general middle-class skepticism toward long-term consumption of allopathic medicines and a belief that they carry side effects, individuals from the professional middle-class segment often turn to homeopathy to address chronic issues or symptoms that are not recognized by allopathy. Hormonal contraceptives in particular generate mistrust and skepticism; as mentioned in Chapter 2, they are thought to negatively affect fertility and overall wellness. Not only do women themselves avoid relying on hormonal contraceptives, but their relatives, friends, and well-wishers also advise women against them.[7] For example, when friends or interlocutors found out I was on oral contraceptives for my PCOS, they would tell me to avoid "taking hormones." So relentless was the dissuading that would follow that I was tempted to prevaricate regarding that aspect of the management of my condition. These conversations frequently led to a recommendation that I try homeopathy instead.

Such pharmacophobia meant that women who had received a PCOS diagnosis but were, in the words of one of my homeopath interlocutors, "scared of hormonal treatment," turned to homeopathy. For many of these women, menstrual irregularities in and of themselves were a sign of general ill health, and they hoped homeopathy would address this. In other cases, they wished to target their hirsutism and hair loss, or, in fewer cases, subfertility issues. Homeopathy was seen as a long-term therapy that was slower in yielding results than allopathy, and women were told by homeopaths to think in terms of months or years rather than weeks in evaluating efficacy. On the other hand, I was told that homeopathy—unlike allopathy and Ayurveda—treated PCOS as a curable condition. This was a stance put forth by my interlocutors with PCOS who were undergoing homeopathic treatment as well as by the homeopaths that I interviewed.

Homeopath interlocutors explained to me that although the therapeutic framework and mode of treatment in homeopathy differ quite significantly from those of allopathy, it relies on many of the same diagnostic categories. Homeopathy therefore recognizes PCOS as a condition; however, treatment—as with all homeopathic remedies—depends upon the individual patient's bodily constitution and mental makeup. Treatment is calibrated to the individual and her constitution. Medication, in the form of homeopathic remedies, is the primary mode of treatment. Nonetheless, some of my homeopath interlocutors did mention the need for their medication to be supplemented with dietary changes and lifestyle interventions. They therefore asked their patients to incorporate stable meal times, regularity in sleep cycles, and light exercise into their daily routines.

Vaidya

Women with PCOS would generally consult *vaidya* after having tried a number of biomedical treatments. As one of my *vaidya* interlocutors put it, they would "come after having roamed and roamed [from doctor to doctor]." Another commented, "Allopathy *karoon yetaat. Kantallele astat.* [They come after having done allopathy. They're tired and fed up]." For *vaidya*, setting expectations with regard to timelines was therefore crucial; women with PCOS were told that they would need to commit to treatment for at least three months, if not longer, to see results.

Vaidya interlocutors revealed that PCOS is not a diagnostic category within Ayurveda. Ayurveda is based on a humoral framework in which individual constitutions are dominated by one or two of the bodily humors of *vata* (wind), *kapha* (mucus), and *pitta* (bile). Illness is thought to result from an imbalance in these humors (Hankey 2005). Moreover, a persistent imbalance in one or more humors is linked to the buildup of *ama* (roughly, metabolic wastes or toxins). The *vaidya* I spoke to explained that the symptoms of PCOS variously fall under Ayurvedic diagnostic categories related to these humors or to *ama*. Individual constitutions and humoral imbalances therefore dictate the treatment course for what allopathy terms PCOS, and there is no standard line of therapy.

Four out of the five *vaidya* I interviewed agreed that PCOS was a *vata* disorder (the fifth thought it resulted from *ama*), but they differed on the specifics. One deemed it to result from *vata* imbalance; another, from an imbalance in both *vata* and *kapha*. The two remaining *vaidya* differentiated between lean PCOS, which they saw as a *vata–pitta* disorder, and PCOS with overweight, which they deemed a *vata–kapha* disorder. The fifth *vaidya*, who linked PCOS to *ama*, said that the phenotypes of PCOS varied based on which humors caused the *ama*.

Of all the practitioners that I interviewed, *vaidya* stressed lifestyle management the most—they recommended changes in diets, meal patterns, sleep times, physical activity, and, in some cases, in clothing (recommending clothing that did not constrict the uterine area). Dietary changes were not limited to calorific restriction alone; certain foods were proscribed and others prescribed, depending upon the humoral imbalance and the potential for certain foods to pacify or aggravate the humors that were out of balance. Treatment could also include *abhyanga*, or massage with imbalance-specific oil infusions. *Vaidya* thus required women to commit significant time and energy resources to treatment, and they emphasized that medication alone, unaccompanied by lifestyle and dietary interventions, would be ineffective.

Practitioners' Perspectives on PCOS

Out of the 30 practitioners that I interviewed, 28 felt that they had seen a rise in the number of PCOS cases in the preceding decade. Of the remaining two, both endocrinologists, one stated that he had not been practicing for long enough to observe a trend (he had been in practice for six years); the other was unable to comment as he was not in a gynecological endocrinology field, which meant that his PCOS patients visited him for comorbidities and complications rather than menstrual irregularities or subfertility alone. Twenty-seven of these practitioners perceived a rise in PCOS cases that they felt could not be attributed to increased awareness and testing alone.

Some of these practitioners' comments are illustrative of the magnitude of the perceived increases in PCOS cases. Dr. Gopalan, a gynecologist, noted that whereas ten years prior he would see about 10–15 PCOS cases in a month, by the time of my fieldwork, that number had shot up to 3–4 cases a day. An endocrinologist who consulted in a government hospital while also working in a private hospital remarked that PCOS prevalence had been "increasing in the last 5–6 years; it's gone up by about 20 per cent." Dr. Sarang, another endocrinologist, found that PCOS levels in India were at epidemic proportions; the high incidence meant, she said, that "PCOS has come out of the closet and onto the coffee table."

Only 3 of these 30 practitioners (a gynecologist, an endocrinologist, and a *vaidya*) thought that PCOS cut equally across class lines. The others perceived it to be higher among the urban middle and upper classes, although some did find it to be on the rise, albeit more slowly, among the lower socioeconomic strata and in rural/peri-urban areas as well. These practitioners' patient bases were not limited to the middle and upper socioeconomic strata; many were consulted by patients from outside these strata, others were consultants in government hospitals that have a predominantly less-than-middle-class base, and a majority were also involved in free medical camps or voluntary initiatives through which they had regular contact with patients from urban and rural low-income groups. Their experience of PCOS cases was therefore not limited to patients from higher socioeconomic strata alone.

Dietary Shifts

As with the media samples and lay epidemiology (Chapter 2), so it was with the medical and paramedical practitioners—a focus on "modern lifestyles" was the norm when it came to explaining the rise in PCOS cases. Modern lifestyles were deemed to include aspects related to diet, a lack of movement, the busy pace of life, stress, and even shifts in gender roles (see Table 4.1). Unlike in lay PCOS epidemiology, where stress was the most cited contributory factor, all medical interlocutors honed in on changing dietary patterns as the main culprit. They blamed eating out, fast food and junk food, the lack of a nutritionally balanced diet, calorie-dense or processed foods, and calorific excess resulting from increased prosperity. Several practitioners recommended a return to older Indian eating habits—a *thali* (plate) with a balanced meal composed of *roti*/rice, vegetables, and legumes, with the proportions of vegetables and legumes increased—and bemoaned the preponderance of "noodles, pizzas, burgers," and Indian junk foods such as *wada pao*.[8]

Several practitioners combined observations regarding dietary shifts with comments on sedentary lifestyles and reduced movement. Endocrinologist Dr. Rahane recited a list of factors implicated in PCOS: "changes in diet, lack of exercise, urbanization/Westernization, changes in environment like in transport, luxurious living, no moving around, sitting at the TV, videos." Dr. Keskar, a gynecologist, noted that diet and exercise problems start early on (an aspect also chronicled in Chapter 3):

> I think lifestyle changes are the main cause. The type of foods the people are eating, more of junk food, not a very balanced diet, lack of exercise, too much of sedentary work, like, I see a lot of young girls who are studying, so they are—between the school, tuitions [academic coaching classes]—they have no time for exercise whatsoever. And maybe nowadays we have more of a nuclear family and small families, so I think [there is an] overindulgence by parents in feeding [their children].

Table 4.1 Themes in Medical Practitioners' Views of PCOS

Theme	Endocrinologists	Gynecologists	Dermatologists	Dietitians	Homeopaths	Vaidya	Total
Total	5	5	5	5	5	5	30
Diet	5	5	5	5	5	5	30
Exercise/physical activity	5	5	5	4	5	5	29
Stress	1	3	4	5	1	5	19
Lack of routine	2	1	2	5	3	5	18
Pollution/adulterants	1	-	3	1	-	1	6
Biomedicines	-	-	-	-	-	2	2

Another gynecologist, Dr. Joshi, pointed to the cultural significance of food:

> Food being the epicenter of Indian, uh, how do you call it, how do you say—whatever you want. Food is of the utmost importance. When you go for a picnic also, the food is important, not the place.

Dr. Ranade, a *vaidya*, observed that calorie-dense food was implicated in a vicious cycle: "There is a sedentary life, then they eat rich food—calorie-rich food—then they don't feel like moving."

Asha Parekh, a dietitian, was more vocal in her critique of nutritionally unsound choices, speaking of a move from "*homo sapiens* to *homo junkiens*." Meanwhile, *vaidya* Dr. Sapre recognized the lifestyle compulsions that resulted in an increased reliance on junk food: "There is no availability of [healthy] food; there are no alternatives. People eat out to survive, not for health reasons." She also blamed an "*aaram sanskruti* [culture of physical relaxation]" that led to comfortably middle-class Indians minimizing movement.

In addition to commenting on shifts in the nutritional content of middle-class diets, the *vaidya*, as well as one dietitian, also had other critiques when it came to food habits. Two *vaidya* mentioned that eating "fridge-cold food" or stale food could contribute to the humoral imbalances that Ayurveda linked to PCOS. One dietitian blamed a tendency to eat while watching TV; this, she said, took people's attention away from their food. Her views were echoed by Dr. Dixit, a *vaidya*:

> These days people, even when eating, they sit in front of the TV and eat. Meaning what happens is that there is actually no attentiveness to the food. Food is there, no? That has to be chewed 32 times. That makes a difference. But then you are eating while watching TV or on one side you are working on your laptop and another side you are eating.

Lack of Routine

Changes in the timings of meals were another aspect of shifts in eating habits that were mentioned. These, along with irregular sleeping patterns, were linked to disrupted circadian rhythms, which are the rhythms linking bodily processes to the sleep–wake cycle. Dermatologist Dr. Fernandes explained that not eating or sleeping on time led to a disturbed body clock, which in turn affected the regularity of the menstrual cycle and hormonal health. Others, such as the endocrinologist Dr. Prasad, connected new communications technologies to such disruptions: "Nowadays teenagers have a lot of distractions. They are constantly getting engaged because of internet and social media like Facebook." As a result of these constant stimulations, he felt, people were unable to fully relax. Homeopath Dr. Shah recommended "adhering the body clock to the clock outside." He added, "They must manage the rhythm of sleep, of meals. Time of sleep is important—I tell patients, 'Don't sleep between sunrise and sunset'." Dr. Arora was even more direct, saying that PCOS was about a "loss of rhythm." Dr. Sapre echoed this view: "Circadian cycle is disturbed; that is main, important in PCOS." By "late sleeping, not eating at regular times, working at times of rest," individuals "waste dopamine [a hormone and neurotransmitter linked to sleep]," leading to endocrine issues. Two other *vaidya* even observed that PCOS was very common among women working in business process outsourcing or information technology jobs because their work occurred on US or European time. This, they felt, led to an upended sleep–wake cycle.

Stress

Medical practitioners, like lay interlocutors, recognized the various pressures experienced by women. Dermatologist Dr. Desai elaborated:

> What happens is, when you're living in a city like Bombay [Mumbai], the day-to-day life is also quite stressful and specially for women. Cause they are managing home, and they are managing outside. And there is a lot of peer pressure, there is a lot of pressure regards *ki* [to] work, and in India, of course, work is totally done by the woman, nobody is going to share the work, the household work. And then they are earning also—I mean the financial aspect and the work outside is of course also there, so it's double work. That is a lot of stress. It's not only women. Even the girls I see, I think the stress in the teenage population is also quite high. That goes for both boys and girls, but girls then get PCOD, whereas boys would probably only manifest only as acne and hair loss—male pattern hair loss also I'm seeing very early.

Several practitioners mentioned the high levels of educational and examination stress faced by adolescents. For example, Dr. Keskar, a gynecologist, said, "Students are under stress of studying, stress of completing their this-thing [studies], so stress can be of any kind—acute levels." Another dimension was of the stress caused by increased aspirations and expectations. Dietitian Asha Parekh called this "self-stress." *Vaidya* Dr. Sapre summed up much of this perspective:

> Priorities have changed. Happy-go-lucky mentality, now no one has that mentality. Nowadays there is an attitude of "even more"....
> For the HPO [hypothalamic—pituitary—ovarian] axis, spirituality, emotions, mind—they have a lot of role in this kind of thing. Mind and uterus is connected through the axis.... Because of the attitude and ambition these days, the frustration level has gone up.

Now women are determined, planning, practical. This is not necessarily bad; earlier they were emotionally fools. Now they are more
determined, but there is some kind of frustration. They can't match
with their ambition; there is less satisfaction.

Two dermatologists also spoke of such stress in terms of most of their
patients having type-A personalities, which are associated with ambition
and impatience. Dermatologist Dr. Fernandes elaborated, "Women want to
excel but they have very little time for everything—they have to do more
than they can. Their aggression fuels testosterone, which then energizes
these traits." This notion of "self-stress" was similar to some of the stress
of increased aspiration that lay interlocutors also mentioned (Chapter 2).
However, Dr. Fernandes was connecting these raised demands from the
self to a feedback loop by which societal expectations, behavior and practices, hormones, and individual aspirations were locked together. Thus, she
suggested, changing gender expectations resulted in women being encouraged to seek careers, but they were still required to shoulder the burden of
managing the household. This forced women to be aggressive in juggling
their workloads; their bodies then aided their aspirations by producing the
testosterone needed to shoulder these overflowing workloads. In essence,
Dr. Fernandes's argument saw PCOS as a form of "biolooping," by which
cultural practices, behaviors, and biological outcomes continuously and
cumulatively interact with and even amplify each other (Hacking 1999).

Notably, two (male) homeopaths also linked PCOS to aggression but saw
this as a process of the "masculinization" of women's behaviors and thought
patterns. Dr. Shah hypothesized that PCOS was the result of women "following the male pattern that is too aggressive, too dominating." He connected this to fertility issues. Management of PCOS, he believed, therefore
required women's "acceptance of their femininity." Similarly, Dr. Arora
believed that PCOS was the result "a female not behaving in a typically
feminine way." For these two homeopaths, PCOS was the body's way of
critiquing a defective modernization that was leveling gender differences.

Pollution, Contamination, and Adulteration

Four biomedical interlocutors held pollution and food additives responsible
for endocrine disruption. Endocrinologist and research scientist Dr. Sarang
was the most vocal: "The environment is nowadays filled with endocrine
disruptors. Plastic bottles, pollution—it is all petrochemicals!" Dr. Patel,
a dermatologist, expressed concern about food additives and pesticides
when it came to hormonal health; two other dermatologists specifically
mentioned hormones in dairy. For example, Dr. Matondkar stated, "Cows
are injected with hormones; chicken has hormones. You go to the villages
and see; they inject prolactin into the cows for more milk." Nonbiomedical
practitioners also spoke of hormones in dairy and "chemicals" in food

(see also Pathak 2020 for more on this discourse on "chemicals") and recommended organic foods for being unadulterated by pesticides and toxicants. Finally, two *vaidya* also spoke of an easy reliance on biomedicine, which led to disturbances in bodily processes and bodily ecology.

Thus, practitioners mentioned a range of factors as contributing to the development of PCOS. Many of these factors were mirrored in the reasons expounded by lay interlocutors. Overall, practitioners blamed faulty diet and exercise patterns far more than the stress that was emphasized by the lay epidemiology of PCOS. Nonetheless, no real pattern related to branches of specialization emerged from practitioners' views. There was, however, a notable pattern in terms of language use. My interviews with biomedical practitioners relied primarily on English, with far fewer switches into Hindi or Marathi than occurred during my interviews with lay interlocutors. There was, on the other hand, much more code-switching between these languages in some of my interviews with *vaidya* and dietitians. This suggests that my biomedical and homeopathic interlocutors, who were trained in English as the language of (Western) science, relied far more exclusively upon English in professional settings. This contrasted with the *vaidya*, who were trained through the use of Sanskrit terms, or dietitians, whose training was not as always as professionalized as that of the other medical practitioners. This dimension of training and expertise bears closer scrutiny.

Medical Objectivity and Medical Subjectivity

As detailed earlier, during the colonial period, the project of modernity was used by the British to justify their rule of India. Science and medicine, indelibly bound up with notions of modernity, were harnessed as instruments of empire and signs of the universal reason accessed by the "West." The British Empire used the pretext of making science and medicine available to their colonial subjects as a key legitimating strategy. Reacting to this framing, the Indian nationalist movement defined a national identity that emphasized India's autonomy from the colonial power and the richness of its traditions (Chatterjee 1993; Prakash 1999; van der Veer 2001). Nevertheless, the colonizer's power was seen to reside in modernity. The result was a discursive conundrum; even as Indian nationalism "challenged the colonial claim to political domination, it also accepted the very intellectual premises of 'modernity' on which colonial domination was based" (Chatterjee 1986: 30). In terms of science, this conundrum led to Indian scientists selectively drawing upon elements of "tradition" to construct an "Indian modernity" (Arnold 2000). Furthermore, the Western-educated Indian elite redefined the authority of science and incorporated it into their own hegemonic project; they positioned themselves as agents of transformation that could mediate between the colonial rulers and the uneducated, irrational masses (Prakash 1999). Since then, biomedicine—key to this hegemonic project—has continued to grow in prestige (Jeffery 1988). Biomedical practitioners, especially specialist practitioners, are at the top of the Indian occupational hierarchy, and medicine, along with engineering, is one the most sought-after professions.

In an ethnography of Indian gastroenterologists, Stefan Ecks (2010) described how those specialist practitioners' claims to distinction rested on distancing themselves, as bearers of reason, from their patients, whom they portrayed as superstitious, unscientific, and irrational quasi-children. This division was less a disconnect between the lower and middle or upper classes than it was between cosmopolitan professionals participating in global circuits of rationality and a localized group of less "enlightened" members of society.

A similar divide was also apparent in my interviews with medical interlocutors. Biomedical practitioners in particular seemed to suggest that their patients showed a flawed modernity that had led to behaviors and practices (such as a reliance on junk food and a reluctance to exercise) that were negatively affecting their health. Just as Ecks's interlocutors fondly distanced themselves from "Bengalis," the biomedical practitioners I interviewed also distanced themselves from "Indians"—by commenting on Indian attitudes to food and sweets and Indians' anxieties regarding "side effects," "chemicals," and medication. Even as they said this, however, they would offer me extremely sweet tea or sweets and cookies. They would mention their reluctance to put teenage patients on hormonal medication or to have women rely on oral contraceptives long term. I would also witness their own disordered and erratic meal times, as they saw patients during standard lunch hours. I do not wish to imply that these practitioners were hypocritical or insincere. Instead, I wish to point out that even as these practitioners, by virtue of their participation in global professional circuits, function as objective commentators on their sociocultural milieu, they are also active participants within that milieu. As specialists in a putatively universal and objective branch of knowledge, their training requires them to cast a critical eye on the very same cultural field in which they are themselves enmeshed. (Indeed, it could be argued that this is not unlike the author, a "native" anthropologist and a participant–observer in her own sociocultural world.)

The matter of genetic susceptibility is also interesting. As described in Chapter 3, Indians are considered metabolically obese even at BMIs that are conventionally considered nonobese. Nonetheless, only 11 of the practitioners I spoke to mentioned a genetic predisposition to metabolic syndrome disorders (three endocrinologists, one gynecologist, three dietitians, one homeopath, and three *vaidya*); this too was just a cursory mention at best. Studies have emphasized how arguments about a genetic predisposition to diabetes and metabolic syndrome disorders are often used to construct Native American and aboriginal populations as diseased and racialized others (e.g., Fee 2006; McDermott 1998; Montoya 2007). However, in my interviews with practitioners, I could not find such a theme. Whereas genetic susceptibility could not be linked to a rise in PCOS cases as such, given that this susceptibility is not novel to the last couple of decades when PCOS numbers have been increasing, it is nonetheless surprising that it was not brought up at all. The focus instead was on lifestyle factors, particularly ones that marked a significant divergence from older patterns of eating and living. PCOS was presented almost as a colonization of Indian ways of living by "modern" practices, as evidenced in multiple mentions of "modern lifestyles." Given that my medical interlocutors were all Indians, this is perhaps unsurprising. It could even be argued that Indians, who are globally extremely well represented in biomedicine, cannot really be classed as its other. Regardless, this speaks to my interlocutors' positionality; despite the objective stance instilled in them as global professional specialists, they did not—or could not—distance themselves so thoroughly from the objects of their clinical gaze.

Medical Individualism

Practitioners' reactions also reflect the changing realities of healthcare in India. Since 1991, with rising affluence and more liberal economic policies allowing for easier importation of medical technology, there has been a rise in healthcare provision in India (Nichter and Van Sickle 2002). Nursing homes and small private hospitals have burgeoned in number. Their patient base is not limited to the middle and upper classes but includes members of the lower classes who are skeptical of the quality of government health services.[9] In addition, there has been a rise in medical diagnostic centers since the 1990s:

> These centres mushroomed in all larger cities and are increasingly found in smaller towns, too. They typically advertise all the diagnostic techniques on offer on billboards visible from the road, making up long lists of acronyms such as MRI (magnet resonance imaging) or CAT (computed axial tomography). Patients usually come to these centres by referral from a doctor to get particular tests done, but sometimes also go directly to a centre of their own choice. In the patients' perspective, "getting a test" goes beyond a regular consultation with a doctor and can signal to family and friends that "something serious" is going on. A test from a lab is seen as much more objective than the impromptu diagnosis done in a doctor's chamber. Indeed, to benefit from the power of visualization, healers of all medical specializations [such as Ayurveda and homeopathy] nowadays refer their patients to these labs.
> (Ecks 2010: 118)

Besides diagnostic testing, there is more use of an increased array of medical resources. People have lower thresholds for discomfort, as they rely more and more on medicines (Nichter and van Sickle 2002). A relaxation in import duties and the easy availability of bank loans have allowed for access to the latest capital-intensive medical technologies such as those used in laser treatments, assisted reproduction, or specialized surgery. New aspects of life are being medicalized—that is, they are being defined and treated through a medical lens (Conrad 1992). The most prominent example of such medicalization is in terms of cosmetic treatments. Previously the preserve of the beauty and personal care industry, cosmetic treatments now overlap with medical treatments (see also Chapters 5 and 6). As mentioned in the earlier chapters, although there has been an increase in life expectancy in India, there has also been a rise in chronic conditions such as type II diabetes and metabolic syndrome disorders. With decreasing mortality rates, individuals live longer, but the increased prevalence of chronic diseases and the greater use of diagnostic testing have, taken together, led to the medicalization of future quality of life. As a result, there has been a turn toward a focus on harm reduction and on reducing the risks of future morbidity. Products and services targeting harm reduction and optimal wellness—such as nutritional supplements, organic food options, protein powders, dietitians, fitness instructors, and yoga classes—have become common.

These two trends are also evident in the medical management of PCOS, where the focus for practitioners is twofold: (1) alleviating PCOS symptoms and (2) mitigating the health risks, such as those of infertility, type II diabetes, and cardiovascular disease, associated with PCOS. In the management of PCOS, symptom alleviation revolved around restoring regular menstruation and addressing cosmetic concerns. Although irregular menstrual cycles have always caused concern and been the objects of medical intervention (see Chapter 2), broad-based resort to medication and medical technology for appearance-related issues, such as those of acne, hirsutism, or hair loss, is a fairly recent development. Historically, beauty work was largely frowned upon by the middle class; such work was sanctioned only around the time when young women started seeking marriage alliances. The last couple of decades have, however, seen a shift toward the greater acceptance of beauty work, with a rise in the expectation that individuals invest effort into improving their appearance to be "presentable" (Pathak 2014).

The focus on the future and risks is also a distinctly modern phenomenon. Theorists from the "risk society" school of thought have argued that modernity brings with it a greater attention to risk (Beck 1989, 1992, 1999; Giddens 1990, 1991, 1999). Anthony Giddens describes the modern era as one of "a society increasingly preoccupied with the future (and also with safety), which generates the notion of risk" (1999: 3). In the field of health, this means that a significant portion of medical management goes beyond alleviating present distress to also emphasize mitigating or preventing a deterioration in future quality of life. Chronic conditions, such as PCOS, are recast as risk states, and their successful management is tied to reducing the potential for anticipated negative developments (Aronowitz 2009).

Although my medical interlocutors recognized large-scale political–economic and sociocultural shifts in the rise in the prevalence of PCOS, they attributed the responsibility of managing the future risks brought by the condition to individual women. Women were expected to work toward lessening those risks, especially in the case of overweight or obese patients. Patients were asked to eat a more balanced diet, incorporate physical activity into their schedules, introduce more structure into their daily routines, or practice stress management techniques; as described, advice varied depending upon the practitioner. Nevertheless, practitioners told me that most women with PCOS were unable to successfully manage their condition. Endocrinologist Dr. Basu said that "there were always excuses" for not making lifestyle interventions; others mentioned only around "30–40 per cent" to "less than ten per cent" of women managed such changes. Moreover, even if and when introduced, these changes were difficult to sustain. Patients' motivation levels fluctuated, resulting in what Dr. Basu called "U-turns"; women would lose excess weight through exercise and dietary interventions when preparing for marriage or conception, but their enthusiasm would wane afterward.

Practitioners acknowledged the difficulties of sustaining healthier lifestyles. Several even spoke of trying to help their patients find ways to make the required interventions. However, none of them could move beyond the individual as the unit of health. Not a single one of my practitioner interlocutors mentioned advising household-level change. Instead, just as in the comments from lay interlocutors (Chapter 2), laments about women's inability to prioritize their health were common. For example, Dr. Sapre commented about women from the middle class that "health *la* last number *detaat* [give the last number (priority) to health]." Dietitian Shilpa Shetty stated, "Nowadays, health is, health is no more a priority. Even I have realized that attitude toward health is a very, very negligent kind of thing."

Elizabeth Fee and Nancy Krieger have written about a tendency within biomedicine to emphasize the biological determinants of illness that prove conducive to healthcare interventions while downplaying, if not outright ignoring, social determinants:

> As several critics have argued, 20th century biomedical models typically are reductionist; they put primacy on explanations of disease etiology that fall within the purview medical intervention narrowly construed, focused on disease mechanisms, and view social factors leading to disease as being secondary, if not irrelevant.... Despite lip service to multifactorial etiology, they seek parsimonious biomedical explanations highlighting the role of one or more proximate agents, and they generally assume that biomedical interventions, operating on biological mechanisms, will be sufficient to control disease.

The biomedical model is also premised on the ideology of individualism. Adopting the notion of the abstract individual from liberal political and economic theory, it considers individuals "free" to "choose" health behaviors. It treats people as consumers who make free choices in the marketplace of products and behaviors, and it generally ignores the role of industry, agribusiness, and governments in structuring the array of risk factors that individuals are supposed to avoid. There is little place for understanding how behaviors are related to social conditions and constraints or how communities shape individuals' lives.

(Fee and Krieger 1993: 1481)

Some of the medical practitioners I spoke to, such as endocrinologist Dr. Sarang, tried to highlight the need for public health action with regard to PCOS, and others tried to include women's mothers or spouses in consultations regarding lifestyle interventions.[10] Nevertheless, for my biomedical and paramedical interlocutors, their training within the individualistic framework described by Fee and Krieger led to an inability to offer therapeutic suggestions that went beyond individual management advice. The practice of biomedicine required them to place the responsibility of management and behavior change upon individual women, even as they recognized their patients' toxic location at the interface of the myriad structural factors that rendered them vulnerable to PCOS.

Intriguingly, this sort of individualism was also in evidence among the nonbiomedical practitioners of homeopathy and Ayurveda. This was despite the fact that Ayurveda in particular recognizes the complicity of social and environmental factors in illness experience. These practitioners were not trained within the biomedical model, but they still emphasized the individual. Thus, all health practitioners, whether biomedical, nonbiomedical, or paramedical, helped naturalize lifestyle disorders as conditions that were within the individual's ultimate realm of control while obscuring the structural factors implicated in the production of their ill health and the management of their condition. A combination of this medical individualism and the medical objectivity described in the earlier section had implications in terms of constraints to PCOS management that arose from the clinical encounter.

The Clinical Encounter and Barriers to Management

Practitioners' focus on the individual meant that the role of the household and social relations in the production of health often went unnoticed and unaddressed. PCOS is strongly tied to the presence of type II diabetes in a first-rank relative; 19 out of 30 of my core interlocutors with PCOS had a parent with diabetes; 4 had parents who were both diagnosed with diabetes.

This familial link suggests that interventions targeting the entire household are crucial not just to women's management of the syndrome but also for the metabolic health of the entire family. Most women found it extremely difficult to make dietary changes for themselves when household eating patterns remained reliant on calorie-dense foods. It created a constant environment of temptation, and resisting temptation then required very high levels of discipline and motivation from women. Moreover, as interlocutor comments in Chapter 3 demonstrate, women were not necessarily the primary decision-makers regarding what was cooked within the home—children, parents-in-law, spouses, and parents had to be considered.

This was compounded by cultural norms governing food and sociality. In India, food is an idiom through which caring, prosperity, and auspiciousness are expressed, and it is one of the few socially sanctioned sources of hedonistic pleasure among the middle class (Wilson 2010). Family members, friends, and even colleagues constantly coax people to eat. For example, an interlocutor with PCOS said of her parents, "you know how Punjabis are—they tell me 'khao, ghee khao, prantha khao [eat, eat clarified butter, eat paratha]'." Another lean interlocutor with PCOS spoke of a double bind when it came to watching her weight to avoid worsening PCOS outcomes: "My friends will say 'Tu toh itni patli hain; tu kyoon nahin kha rahin? [You are so thin; why are you not eating?]'." If she did not watch what she ate, she would put on weight and worsen her PCOS, but as she was not putting on weight, her friends and family thought she need not watch what she ate.

Such coaxing is especially pronounced when it comes to sweets, which are symbols of auspiciousness and festivity. Refusing sweets, especially during celebrations or festivals, is comment-worthy and usually deemed rude, selfish, or uptight. Given that the festival season in a diverse, cosmopolitan environment such as that of Mumbai lasts around mid-August through December (the heterogeneity of residents means that festivals from various communities become occasions for celebration),[11] this becomes a tricky situation to navigate. As mentioned earlier, even when I met with healthcare professionals, I was offered sugary tea and sweets. Again, this is not a critique of the practitioners—they were being gracious in following norms of hospitality—but rather to point to the wider sociocultural context that valorizes food and sweets. In such a context, health-related advice that is tailored to individual action while neglecting the role of the household and family members is in itself a barrier to management.

The focus on the individual, combined with the numerous constraints to individual behavior change, meant that practitioners would often assume that women would not seriously commit to dietary or lifestyle interventions. At the same time, given the time pressures on practitioners, consultations were often too short for elaborate communication. Only a handful of my interlocutors with PCOS recalled being told of the increased risks of type II diabetes and cardiovascular disease by their doctors. Practitioners were thus either failing to provide this information (although in my interviews, most claimed otherwise), or they were doing so in a manner that was not aiding comprehension and retention. Many of my interlocutors reported that the lifestyle advice their doctors provided was only an admonition to exercise, eat healthier, or lose weight. What exactly constituted exercise (for example, in India even a daily nonbrisk walk is often glossed as exercise) or a healthier diet was not elaborated upon. Conversations with women with PCOS along with interviews with practitioners suggested that practitioners were largely relying on the paternalistic "classic relationship" communication model (Stokken 2009). In such a model, patients are seen to lack knowledge and are expected to follow the doctor's orders unquestioningly. Within such a relationship, there is no room for patients to express concerns regarding management advice.

With the widespread penetration of the internet, women had access to a deluge of PCOS-related information. They found sifting through this material and filtering out what was relevant to them scary and confusing. Furthermore, they would receive a range of opinions on their condition from a set of people as diverse as family members, friends, colleagues, acquaintances, or staff in pharmacies, beauty salons, and other shops. In India, knowledge perceived to stem from experience carries an authority that technomedical expertise has not displaced. Health advice is therefore not the sole preserve of experts, and offering opinions on health—even to relative strangers—is acceptable practice. As a dermatologist that I interviewed rather drily remarked, "Here in India, there are a lot of doctors nearby. All your neighbors are doctors. And all grannies are also doctors; mothers are also doctors." People are constantly commenting on health matters, and they are not loath to contest advice from medical practitioners.

When women with PCOS thought that their medical practitioners were not sufficiently engaging with them and their concerns regarding management, they found it a struggle to determine what information to trust. Furthermore, interlocutors were very suspicious of hormonal contraceptives and insulin sensitizers, which were seen as "strong" medicines that have deleterious long-term effects. Women were frequently told by relatives and friends that these medications were harmful, or they would be informed by staff at pharmacies that they had been prescribed "diabetes medicine." In such cases, especially when their doctors had not explained the need for these drugs to their satisfaction, women became even more skeptical and anxious. They then found themselves with questions that they did not know how to get addressed. The case of one interlocutor is revealing here. She told me that when she was diagnosed with PCOS, her gynecologist had merely written out a prescription for medication; he had not explained the condition, its risks, or how to manage those risks. The interlocutor had queries, but the gynecologist's attitude precluded getting them answered. She was still largely in the dark when we spoke, and she ended up asking me for clarification on the syndrome. This was not rare; I often found myself answering queries from women with PCOS regarding the condition and its management, queries that practitioners had apparently failed to address. Unsurprisingly, then, I found that the women who felt most comfortable talking to their doctors and getting their queries answered were also more likely to successfully implement some degree of dietary and lifestyle changes.

Furthermore, gynecologists' and endocrinologists' attitudes toward overweight and obese women were often insensitive, and overweight interlocutors with PCOS spoke of feeling fat shamed. In an interview, for example, a gynecologist mentioned telling one of her patients that even if she didn't eat for a week, she would be fine. One of my interlocutors with PCOS was at the receiving end of such a comment; she was told at her visit to an endocrinologist to "only come back" for her next consultation if she lost weight. Rather than spurring her to action, it made the issue of weight loss a shame-laden one, turning her away from making dietary or movement-related changes. When it came to weight loss, another relatively slim interlocutor with PCOS was told by her gynecologist to lose a few kilograms to help her conceive. The gynecologist offered no explanation, and the interlocutor, who was not visibly overweight, was puzzled and offended by the advice.

This feeling of not being heard or respected led women to consult several doctors before settling on one that they trusted (if at all). In the absence of substantive patient–practitioner communication, they treated the medical advice they received as suspect, often avoiding follow-ups or starting and stopped prescription medication without supervision. Such unsupervised consumption of medicines can adversely affect PCOS symptoms, whether menstruation, hirsutism, or weight gain. In women with PCOS and insulin resistance, it can also result in uncontrolled blood sugar levels, hypoglycemia (low blood sugar), and hyperglycemia (elevated blood sugar), which can all cause organ damage over the long term.

Women's skepticism was exacerbated by a lack of consensus among medical practitioners. A study from Australia reported differences between gynecologists and endocrinologists in PCOS diagnosis and management (Cussons et al. 2005), and I found an even more marked difference in the Indian context. Endocrinologists treated PCOS as a hormonal disorder and handled it as a diagnosis of exclusion, requiring myriad diagnostic tests to rule out complications. Moreover, they were the only practitioners who regularly mentioned increased risks of type II diabetes, hypertension, and cardiovascular disease to patients. Meanwhile, gynecologists tended to treat PCOS as a menstrual/reproductive disorder. Not all gynecologists required hormonal assays or tests to rule out complications, and in many cases, they delivered a diagnosis on the basis of a sonography and clinical symptoms alone. A few asked overweight or obese patients to undergo glucose tolerance tests in the case of suspected insulin resistance. Some gynecologists even prescribed insulin sensitizers without testing for insulin resistance, on the basis of overweight or obesity alone. Furthermore, gynecologists' focus was on reproductive health, and I heard of them advising women not to be concerned about PCOS unless in relation to conception. Gynecologists were also less likely to inform patients of the link between PCOS and increased risks of type II diabetes and other metabolic manifestations.

There were similar differences in the treatment approaches and health advice offered by other practitioners. As mentioned, dietitians can practice in India with just a post-graduate diploma and need not have experience in dietetics linked to the medical management of chronic conditions. As a result, they offer a range of advice, often contradictory, depending upon their experience and qualifications. Meanwhile, homeopaths tell women that PCOS is curable (unlike biomedical practitioners and *vaidya*), and *vaidya* insist upon a commitment to lifestyle changes that go beyond calorie restriction and increased physical activity. These contradictory diagnostic and management techniques mean that women with PCOS get very different advice depending upon which specialists they visit. This not only makes it difficult to learn how to successfully manage the condition, but it also contributes to a trust deficit in the healthcare profession overall.

Here, it is also worth highlighting a dependence upon overweight as a symptom. Medical practitioners pointed out that most women with PCOS in India have issues with overweight or obesity. However, the reliance on overweight or obesity as a clinical marker of PCOS causes practitioners to miss out on cases of lean PCOS. A slim woman with PCOS myself, I was only diagnosed in my late 20s by my dermatologist, whom I consulted for stubborn cystic acne that kept getting worse with age. Prior to that, I had repeatedly complained to various medical practitioners, including gynecologists, regarding heavy and troublesome menstrual periods, but I found that my concerns were usually dismissed as stemming from anemia or a low threshold for pain. The possibility that I may have PCOS was never considered, and I was repeatedly recommended iron supplements and dissuaded from exploring hormonal contraceptives. I heard from one of my interlocutors with lean PCOS that she too had very painful, heavy periods, but her distress had been ignored by her doctors. In conversations about menstrual issues with women in Mumbai—not all of whom suffered from PCOS—I learned that complaints regarding heavy bleeding and painful periods were seldom taken seriously by practitioners. Studies have documented a bias in treatment such that women's pain (compared to men's) is habitually downplayed in the clinical encounter (e.g., Samulowitz et al. 2018), and fieldwork revealed that when it came to PCOS, women's subjective experiences of distress were devalued in favor of visible symptoms. Again, this not only eroded women's trust in the healthcare profession, but it also impeded early diagnosis and successful management outcomes.

Clinical Encounters with PCOS

Given its wide range of symptoms, PCOS involves contact with several medical and paramedical practitioners for diagnosis and management. In this chapter, I examined such contact and the common trajectories that it followed across life stages. Women's contact with healthcare practitioners reflects wider changes in the Indian healthcare landscape, with a shift toward a higher incidence of chronic and metabolic disorders, the medicalization of new domains, including cosmetic concerns and future quality of life, and a greater preoccupation with risk and harm reduction.

When speaking of PCOS, medical practitioners recognized the role of large-scale socioeconomic shifts in the sociocultural production of health and spoke of women with PCOS as being caught in a defectively "modern" system that made healthy living difficult. Nonetheless, practitioners were also enmeshed in the very same contexts that they commented upon as professionals in global circuits of technical expertise. Their training within an individual-centered model of intervention also meant that they helped naturalize lifestyle disorders as ultimately residing within the individual's locus of control. Despite acknowledging the complicity of a toxic location in their patients' PCOS, they could not move beyond the individual as the site of healthcare analysis and intervention. This inability meant that the clinical encounter brought with it several barriers to the early diagnosis and effective management of the condition. In the next chapter, I examine women's PCOS-related concerns and their experiences of navigating the condition in the midst of these constraints.

Notes

1 A system of medicine thought to have originated in the South Indian state of Tamil Nadu, very similar to Ayurveda.
2 A humoral system of medicine based on the teachings of Galen and developed further by Arabic and Persian physicians (the word Unani comes from Ionian); seen as a "Muslim" system of medicine.
3 These supplements, while marketed as "Ayurvedic medicines," would more accurately be termed herbal medicines or food supplements. Whereas Ayurveda requires a practitioner to personalize therapies and medication to suit a patient's constitution (symptoms are considered to result from constitutional issues that differ from patient to patient; similar symptoms can be rooted in different underlying issues), these supplements are standardized, mass-marketed, and targeted at various conditions or the optimization of health rather than at problems stemming from individual patient constitutions (see also Bode 2008).
4 There is a tendency in India, especially pronounced among the middle and higher socioeconomic strata, to visit specialists rather than general practitioners or family physicians; visits to hospitals are common even for basic healthcare. The high expenses of a medical education also mean that super specializations are sought at the cost of a basic medical degree, such that there is a dearth of general practitioners in the country. Of all the women with PCOS that I interacted with, none visited a general practitioner, and as I point out later in this chapter, this negatively affected management.
5 It was presumed that women would not be trying to conceive prior to getting married.
6 The glycemic index measures how much a food increases blood sugar levels; low glycemic index foods cause lower increases in blood sugar levels than high glycemic index foods.

7 This appears to be a larger regional phenomenon; Nichter and Nichter (1996) chronicled a similar distrust of oral contraceptives in Sri Lanka.

8 A fried potato patty sandwiched in a white bread bun.

9 Government-run health centers and hospitals provide subsidized, low-cost medical care. Private healthcare costs more, but it is generally perceived to be more reliable and of higher quality (though this need not actually be the case).

10 Women were seldom at the center of family interventions. Whereas the household would adapt its practices to suit the medical advice offered to a husband, parent, or child, as noted in Chapter 3, this was not necessarily the case for a woman once she had stepped into the role of wife or daughter-in-law. Nevertheless, there are some indications that this situation may be changing; see Chapter 5.

11 With celebrations for Janmashtami, the Ganesh festival, Navratri, Dussehra, Diwali, Eid, Christmas, and New Year's Eve, followed by the wedding season.

5

"WHEN YOU ARE 17 OR 18, IT DOESN'T BOTHER YOU"

Living with PCOS

As mentioned in the earlier chapters, India has experienced an accelerated healthcare transition since the liberalization of its economy. The 1980s and 1990s had already witnessed the rapid expansion of the private healthcare segment and corporate healthcare respectively. The Indian government had encouraged the growth of these segments through land subsidies and concessions for the import of technologies, and private and corporate healthcare had been included under government insurance schemes (Baru 2000). Economic liberalization brought further reforms in the health sector; there were cutbacks in the public sector and the simultaneous easing of requirements for privatization and public–private partnerships. In 2002, the Government of India declared urban medical institutions to be service production units and important sources of foreign exchange, and the state started actively promoting the country as a global healthcare provider. Since then, India has emerged as a leading destination for medical tourism (Reddy and Qadeer 2010). Although India banned commercial surrogacy in 2015, it is still a major location for people seeking other reproductive services. The country offers access to cutting-edge reproductive technologies, including assisted reproductive technologies such as IVF, at relatively accessible prices for a global market, and estimates suggest that already in 2010 there were over 3,000 IVF centers across India (Bharadwaj 2000; Gupta 2000; Reddy et al. 2018; Unnithan 2010). Such services are marketed not just to an overseas audience but also to Indians of the upper and comfortably middle classes, including women from the urban professional middle-class segment.

In Chapter 4, I touched upon how this health transition has meant that healthcare practitioners think of conditions such as PCOS as risk states. This brings a focus on harm reduction and the medical management of the future quality of life. How, though, has this affected the lived experiences of women from the urban professional middle class with PCOS? This chapter centers on that question to examine how, for women from this class segment, lived experiences of PCOS are affected by the medicalization of new domains of life and the commodification of health. These experiences, I argue, also reflect new middle-class subjectivities linked to reasonings of risk and probability.

DOI: 10.4324/9781003171423-5

PCOS and Future Health Risks

When I spoke to interlocutors with PCOS, I found that of all the issues linked to their condition, the increased risks of other metabolic syndrome conditions, such as type II diabetes or heart disease, distressed them the least. This is not entirely surprising. Future risks tend to feel less immediate and, therefore, less worth worrying about. As chronicled in Chapter 3, the women I spoke to typically did not, and indeed felt they could not, make the dietary (and less often physical activity-related) modifications that were recommended by their healthcare practitioners; such modifications, besides helping to manage symptoms, are also necessary to mitigate future risks. Instead, I found that the ubiquity of metabolic syndrome disorders in India and the proliferation of medication and other medical interventions to address these disorders had enabled the "commodification of health" (Nichter 1989) among the urban professional middle class. As I go on to describe, this meant that among this class segment, health was treated as a state that could be bought back, through the consumption of appropriate products and services, once it had been degraded. Women were therefore much less concerned with prophylactic action that required them to diligently change their patterns of living.

Concern regarding future risks manifested itself instead more as harm reduction. Harm reduction is a strategy through which individuals try to reduce their sense of vulnerability and provide themselves with a sense of control when it comes to health risks (Nichter 2003). The harm reduction practices that my interlocutors engaged in could not really be attributed to reducing the specific health risks brought by PCOS. They were instead targeted at general wellness. That is, women engaged in practices that they saw as reducing their risks of future conditions, be they type II diabetes or cancer, but they did not mention these practices as being related to their PCOS.

Interlocutors' harm reduction practices largely revolved around consumption. They spoke of using "herbal" or "Ayurvedic" products as they did not have "side effects" or "chemicals." This was especially pronounced when using skincare or cosmetic products that targeted hair fall or acne. Women saw these PCOS symptoms as being aggravated by pollution (see also Chapter 2), and by using products targeting the ill effects of such pollution and environmental contamination, they felt that they were managing threats to appearance as well as to general wellness.

Interlocutors also engaged in practices of "precautionary consumption" (MacKendrick 2010)—that is, they were consuming in ways that are meant to reduce risk. Such practices included eschewing the use of plastics—thought to release harmful chemicals—for storing or heating food, avoiding "nonbranded" food products (which, they believed, were more likely to be adulterated or contaminated), or favoring milk from organic dairies. These practices could be seen to index concerns with environmental pollution and toxicity. Nevertheless, women did not relate these practices directly to the management of their PCOS or even to avoiding EDCs. Precautionary consumption has been shown to be a highly inadequate strategy when it comes to avoiding the health effects of environmental degradation or to preventing exposure to EDCs. It is not possible to insulate oneself to any significant degree from environmental contamination through careful, individualized consumption. Nevertheless, interlocutors did not translate their concern with future risks, exhibited through acts of precautionary consumption, into collective action. This is not atypical; harm reduction practices, by focusing on the individual, often deflect attention and action away from addressing risks at the level of population health (Nichter 2003).

The example of 36-year-old Shruti can prove illuminating here. Shruti's case represented the most extensive degree of action to reduce future health risks of all my interlocutors—she had undergone bariatric surgery. Prior to the surgery, she said, she "was the ideal candidate for cardiac arrest by the age of 35." She had weighed 94 kilograms before her surgery. At her height of 5'2", this yielded a BMI of 38, which is considered morbidly obese. Shruti blamed biomedicine for her PCOS—she believed that taking oral contraceptives for a few days to delay her periods around the time of her wedding had triggered the condition. She also spoke scathingly of several clinical encounters with highly unsympathetic doctors. Nevertheless, she was unfailingly positive about her experience with bariatric surgery. Surgery reduced her future health risks and allowed her to go off the insulin sensitizers that she had been prescribed to manage her PCOS. It also changed the way that people perceived her.

Although the stated aim for Shruti's surgery had been to address her obesity in order to mitigate health risks, it was apparent that the most vivid and tangible results had been in terms of her appearance. Our interactions revealed her great pleasure in her new, slimmer body and the changed social reactions it brought her. She repeatedly spoke of "being hot" and looking like "a model." However, she also distanced herself from that pleasure. She told me that she did not wish to flaunt her body or take comments about her changed appearance as compliments. She did not admit to surgery when people who had seen her dramatically shed weight asked for advice. Instead, she asked them to eat smaller, more frequent meals. This, she told me, was what bariatric surgery ultimately forced one to do anyway. Shruti claimed that she was reluctant to tell people about her surgery because she didn't want to endorse such an intervention to people who might not understand all its costs and risks.

Shruti's case was highly unusual, and it illustrates the difficulties of separating out issues relating to the commodification of health, future health risks, functional health (being healthy enough to comfortably go about one's daily activities), and appearance as they relate to weight. For example, Shruti continued smoking heavily even after her surgery; she would chain smoke throughout all our interactions. The cardiovascular risks of smoking, compounded by PCOS and its metabolic dimensions, did not cause her to quit. Lowering risks, aiding functional health, and enhancing her appearance through the consumption of the expensive medical service of bariatric surgery (expenses for which came to around INR 200,000 or USD 2,800) seemed more achievable.

PCOS and Presentability

The aspect of appearance highlighted in Shruti's story is a significant one. Across ages and life stages, it was the symptoms related to appearance—the weight gain, acne, and hirsutism—that caused women with PCOS the most distress. Sapna, a never-married 29-year-old media professional, told me that "PCOD has changed my life drastically, and all in a bad way." As we talked, I realized that all of the negatives that she was associating with PCOS were related to her appearance. Her periods had been extremely irregular prior to her PCOS diagnosis, but she wasn't bothered by that irregularity. Instead, she was troubled by the "weird boils [cystic acne]" that "would just not go." It had been the acne that had led her to a dermatologist and a PCOS diagnosis. When we first spoke, she was on anti-androgenic medication and hormonal contraceptives. These had not managed to address her acne, and they caused severe mood swings to boot. Nevertheless, Sapna found the cystic acne to be distressing enough that she continued with the medication despite the mood swings. When we met again a few months afterward, her mood swings had improved and the acne was much better controlled. However, she was still bothered by the weight she had gained around her middle. "This portion [pointing to lower stomach] is bulging," she told me. "Otherwise, I'm very thin, but only this portion has started bulging."

Some of my interlocutors related the distress over their appearance to effects on their professional lives. Shruti, who had undergone bariatric surgery, was a public relations professional, and she elaborated:

> I was in public relations, for crying out loud. Image is everything! And I looked like that [obese]. You're battling with the image issue, you're battling with the fact that you don't have children, you're battling with people who are pretty much your age who look like a million bucks and that's what you look like.

Shruti told me that the people she had worked with had assumed that she wasn't competent on the basis of her weight. Besides this, her parents-in-law and husband were unsympathetic, blaming her weight gain on laziness and an inability to stick to her diet. In a similar vein, Monica, a 38-year-old dance fitness instructor, expressed concern that her PCOS was negatively affecting her job. She worried that clients, who typically were looking to lose weight through dance, judged her to be incompetent because of her PCOS-related overweight.

In my interviews with medical practitioners, I had heard similar accounts of how career prospects could be tied to appearance. The dermatologist Dr. Fernandes observed,

> In certain industries, maybe not regular, but in aviation, I've had airhostesses who have been grounded because of pimples or you know whatever. For the regular other jobs—maybe an actress or a model or whatever—but other jobs it doesn't really [matter]— people want to look presentable, so they take the treatment. But it doesn't hamper their jobs, but it helps their self-esteem if the skin is clear.

However, as Dr. Fernandes pointed out, it was difficult to disentangle concerns about external reactions from an embodied sense of self. Forty-three-year-old scientist Sunita explained this in terms of how her body felt to her:

> I'm bigger-boned and people have never said, "You're so fat"…. I am certainly conscious about it. You know, I'm conscious in that I won't wear certain clothing, like, I wouldn't wear a dress or I wouldn't wear a skirt because I just would feel fat in it. Whereas that was not the case when I was much thinner. I won't wear short T-shirts; I'll usually wear longer T-shirts. The minute I get fatter, I start wearing *salwar kameezes*. It's just the reality. It's cause I can't—I don't like the look of my own body. So it's a sense of "Oh yeah, you know what, I'm not happy with my body right now" so it's a sliding scale. Everybody knows that I'm happier with my body because I'm back to my jeans and T-shirts…It's not a "I want to look good" it's a "How do I feel about the way my body feels to me."

Sunita felt most comfortable when she was at the lower end of her BMI range. Weight gain, even when her weight was still within a healthy BMI range, made her feel less like herself. "This doesn't feel like my body," she explained.

Appearance-related concerns were a deep source of anxiety and suffering for interlocutors. One interlocutor who had struggled with acne revealed,

> Around that time I was very—I don't know if I was depressed, but it was certainly how I felt…. I was ready to try on anything that would help…. I was an easy target for anybody selling anything—I would buy.

Her reaction was a common one. For example, 30-year-old Sakshi thought her overweight body frustrated her desires to wear Western wear such as jeans and skirts, and Neha's hirsutism, she felt, stopped her from "dressing up."

My interlocutors' experiences point to changes in appearance-related subjectivities in post-liberalization India. During the colonial period in India, the nationalist movement contrasted a "spiritual" India against a "materialistic" West (Chatterjee 1993). Gender was crucial to this conceptualization, and middle-class women were expected to both perform and preserve an "Indianness" that was linked to tradition and respectability. One of the legacies of this gendered formulation was that a middle-class woman was deemed vain or shallow for showing an interest in her appearance (S 1998; Mazzarella 2003; Munshi 2001). Appearance, especially fairness, was undoubtedly important for women, especially with regard to their marriageability, but an interest in enhancing or working on one's appearance could detract from a woman's respectability. It was generally only sanctioned—and that too in heavily circumscribed ways—when a woman was of "marriageable age" (e.g., Davis 2009).

This changed after economic liberalization, with the relaxation of taxes related to personal care and other products deemed unessential, easier access to previously unavailable beauty-related consumer goods and services, and a surge in aspirational media images and marketing messages. Beauty was commodified to become something that could be achieved through the consumption of goods, such as beauty products and cosmetics, and services, such as personal physical training and cosmetology. Beauty work became not just accepted but also, to a large degree, expected; the turn toward the imperative that individuals work on their appearance to be "presentable" has been a gradual, but definite, trend in India since the 1990s (Pathak 2014).

Writing about neoliberalism, Nikolas Rose has argued that it results in

> an ethic in which the maximization of lifestyle, potential, health, and quality of life has become almost obligatory, and where negative judgments are directed toward those who will not, for whatever reason, adopt an active, informed, positive, and prudent relation to the future.
>
> (Rose 2006: 25)

I have pointed out elsewhere that working on one's appearance in contemporary India is similarly linked to maximizing one's potential:

> Changes following on the heels of economic liberalization allowed individuals the unprecedented freedom to work on their bodies, and therefore, their selves. Not taking this opportunity for improvement is considered irresponsible—comments from my informants included "has she even looked at herself in the mirror?," "look at how he keeps himself!," "*thoda toh karna padega* [you have to do at least a little (on your appearance)]!"—and individuals' inability or disinterest in caring for their appearance is condemned as a

personal failure. With the commodification of beauty, looking good is not just a possibility but also an imperative; everyone not only can, but also should, look good.

(Pathak 2014: 324)

Against this backdrop, presentability is required of prospective employees, service providers, and mates/spouses. This is especially pronounced among the professional middle-class segment. Furthermore, this imperative structures subjectivity by offering new pleasures that invite people to "desire and collude with it" (Eagleton 1990: 37). Thus, the focus on appearance goes beyond concerns about creating good first impressions, whether professional and personal, on others. It becomes linked to affective states, as a source of both pleasure, when one fulfills norms of presentability, and pain, when one cannot.

Meanwhile, body size ideals have also shifted. Prior to the 1990s, the Indian media and Bollywood (and other regional) movies featured women with fuller figures. Well-rounded bodies were normative. Furthermore, body size was typically only a focus around the time of a woman's search for matrimonial prospects; after getting married, and especially after childbirth, women were not expected, indeed even actively discouraged, from putting effort into keeping in shape. However, this has changed with the exposure to global media images of slimmer women, an influx of transnational fashion-related goods and products, and the increased popularity of Western wear, which draws attention to a woman's slimness more than conventional Indian wear does. There has been a move toward a slimmer body ideal, and a greater acceptability of the dieting and exercise required to achieve it (Dhillon and Dhawan 2011; Pathak 2014; Talukdar 2012). This ideal is much more prevalent among the urban professional middle and upper classes, which show a closer engagement with modernity and which tend to be more exposed to global media messages. The women more likely to be affected by PCOS and its associated weight gain are therefore also the women more likely to espouse thinner body preferences.

Both dimensions—the increased focus on appearance and the move to slimmer body ideals—were apparent in the narratives of my interlocutors. Notably, interlocutors spoke only of keeping to the weight they had as late adolescents or young adults rather than of becoming thinner than that. Those who had not been slim adolescents did not seem to aspire to be thinner than they had ever been. Shabina, for example, commented, "See, I was always on the fat side. So, I've never experienced this 'thinner beauty' of a female. I've never, never been on the thin side. I'm not bothered after [about being thin] that experience." Shabina's focus was on preventing further weight gain rather than on being slim per se. Similarly, interlocutors did not speak of dropping dress sizes but rather of being able to fit into their old clothes. Thus, the only interlocutor who said she was not much troubled by the weight gain aspects of her PCOS had been overweight even as a young child.

Addressing PCOS-related weight gain could therefore not be simplistically attributed to interlocutors' desires to conform to new slimmer body ideals. Rather, it was about loss aversion, not wishing to lose the advantages in terms of presentability that they had once had, and a new subjectivity that related appearance to a sense of self. The weight gain that concerned the women I spoke to was that which was in excess of what they considered *normal for themselves*. Their conceptions were undoubtedly influenced by the new body ideals; where slim women may once have welcomed some weight gain, this was now being eschewed as undesirable. Overweight and obese interlocutors, whether single or married, also spoke of their weight in terms of being unable to be as active as they would like and about being unable to engage in activities that they once did without exhaustion. Here again, body weight was tied to a sense of embodied personal identity rather than to aspiration alone.

PCOS and Subfertility

In contrast to the appearance-related symptoms of PCOS, subfertility was not a concern for my interlocutors prior to their getting married and trying to conceive. For example, 32-year-old engineer Priyanka said, about the possibility of infertility, "When you're 18 and 19, it doesn't really bother you." Priyanka had been diagnosed with PCOS as a teenager, and her doctor spoke about PCOS largely in terms of its effects on fertility. Priyanka recalled being relieved by this:

> If that is the only thing that can probably go wrong, meaning me not being able to have a baby, that's okay. But if it does affect my overall health in many different ways, then maybe I would have continued with medication. If the baby was the only question mark, I said I could still live with it.... When I heard that the only thing was I couldn't conceive, I was very happy.

Shabina, the 23-year-old advertising executive mentioned earlier, stated, regarding her possible subfertility, "I don't take *fukat ka* [unnecessary] stress." She thought she might like a child, but at her age—being years away from trying to conceive—her fertility potential did not much preoccupy her. Such a lack of concern was not a product of age alone. Vidya, a gregarious 29-year-old who was not married and not contemplating motherhood, said that when it came to her fertility, "I haven't even thought about it or gone there."

Nevertheless, as women started actively planning pregnancies, PCOS-related subfertility became a cause of distress. Sucheta, aged 32, started trying to conceive a couple of years after getting married. When meeting prospective spouses through arranged marriage channels, she had brought up the possibility of subfertility and childlessness with the men. She had felt ready to face whatever the future would bring. Faced with the tangible possibility of infertility, however, she was shaken:

> I had some idea [about the possibility of PCOS], but *fir bhi* [even then] when it actually falls on you, you take some time to get out of it *ki* [that] it may happen, that chance. Till today I was only thinking that it could happen, and it was actually happening.... there was a phase of almost a month when I was very depressed because I was only thinking about this. I would think about "Oh shit! I will have to go for IVF"—a hundred things would come into my mind.

The experience of Sunita, the scientist mentioned earlier, mirrored that of Sucheta. It echoed many of the themes recounted by other interlocutors—subfertility initially not being a concern, the desire to have a child after years of delaying childbearing, trying to get pregnant, and the depression that followed every menstrual period as it signaled a lack of conception:

> When I was 32 was when I first felt like I really want to have a baby. So I was 32, I told Siddharth [her husband] that I really want to have a baby, but he was like "Uhh, no, I'm not sure," etc. And then I went into a busy stage again, so we didn't really seriously try at 32. But when I was 33, I knew by the time that I really want a kid now. And I didn't want to wait, at that point in time, to find out if I was going to be naturally fertile or not ... [the gynecologist] put me on clomiphene [ovulation inducer]. I did two cycles of Clomid [clomiphene], and neither was successful, and I wept buckets because it did a real number on my nervous system because I didn't realize how that hormonal flux was going to get me down. I mean, I did two cycles, and I remember my second cycle, getting my period and going to the loo—and the minute I got my period, I would start crying. I think in my mind, I knew that there is an infertility component to PCOS, so because I knew that I took every cycle as "Oh my God!" you know?

Similarly, Shruti spoke of her unhappiness as she watched her friends get pregnant while she was desperately trying to conceive. Seeing them successfully undertake a life phase that she felt excluded from exacerbated her deep-seated desire for a child and caused her considerable anguish.

Interlocutor narratives highlighted the fact that concerns about fertility were linked to life stage. Although fertility is often not a concern for women of the professional middle-class segment until they start trying to conceive, this can change once they start anticipating childbearing. At this point, when conception takes longer than they expected and they see others around them successfully getting pregnant, the possibility of childlessness becomes a source of significant anxiety.

The Materiality of the Body

Medical anthropology has long acknowledged that the materiality of the body can aid or constrain the aspirations of the self. Even though my interlocutors did not report feeling like "freaks" or not "proper women" as did the UK-based women with PCOS that were interviewed by Celia Kitzinger and Jo Willmott (2002), their narratives reveal how PCOS nevertheless formed a "visible identity" (Alcoff 2006) that was anchored in their physical bodies. PCOS-related symptoms formed barriers to their desires to be presentable subjects, to wear certain kinds of clothes, and to create favorable first impressions. As they tried to conceive, PCOS-related subfertility also loomed large as a threat to their desire to be mothers. Their disordered bodies had the potential to thwart their aspirations and disrupt their identities.

What, however, about possibly aiding their aspirations? Sunita, the neurobiologist, had an intriguing hypothesis. She suggested that PCOS might confer upon women an adaptive advantage in a hypercompetitive environment:

One thing I read about is whether women who are achievers and are driven might be slightly prone to [PCOS]—I think it's a question like chicken and egg. Because you are PCOS you become slightly more driven because your testosterone is slightly higher than other women, and whether that gives you a certain competitive or an aggressive edge, I don't know.... I've always wondered whether we are sub-selecting out a pool of women who now, because of the environmental circumstances, their PCOS might actually become an advantage for them in their environment. I mean, at some level maybe that elevated testosterone gives you a certain advantage in the workspace. Our workspace is very patriarchal, and we are driven to looking toward women—at least quiet, demure women—very differently from women who have an opinion and who speak up. I wonder—I mean this is hypothetical, a completely arbitrary argument.

Sunita went on to connect this to an urban environment contaminated with EDCs:

I also know that there must be environmental estrogens around, quite a few of them, xenoestrogens which fool your body into constantly feeling stimulated by hormones and that might then cause this sort of a situation.... Environmental estrogens change the programming of your gonadal axis. So your body sees a lot of estrogens. Xenoestrogens and estrogens anyway can bind to testosterone and androgen receptors because they can cross. I think your body is constantly faced with these at an early age, I mean it is programmed to—I mean, why suddenly and why urban women more than rural women? If it's just an environment thing, is it only an environment that urban women are exposed to and not rural women? It's not very clear. Also, I feel, it would be very interesting to ask the number of women who have polycystic ovarian syndrome and how they have done in their careers versus not. I wonder if our systems are such that it's providing almost a selection advantage. Is there some advantage to having slightly elevated— slightly elevated so you don't move into the zone of testosterone where you "turn-into-a-male" like place, but it takes you a notch over what your average woman would have.

In my interviews with medical practitioners (Chapter 4), I had heard similar arguments linking PCOS, as a bodily result, to changes in gender norms, expectations, and pressures. Similarly, two of my interlocutors with PCOS jokingly suggested that they were more aggressive because of their PCOS-linked higher testosterone levels. If PCOS had the potential to constrain some dimensions of identity and aspiration, could it also be simultaneously aiding the pursuit of other identities? The question of whether the higher androgenic activity of PCOS can really convey a selective advantage and whether higher androgens can even be linked to assertiveness in such a straightforward manner is one that I cannot answer; I have neither the requisite expertise nor the data to do so. However, setting aside that question, these interlocutors' views offer a tantalizing hypothesis on how social norms and gender performances come to be materialized, or what Judith Butler (1990, 1993) terms "congealed," at the site of the body. Their views offer glimpses into how gender norms hold the potential to mold the body such that those very same gender norms in turn seem "natural." They also highlight the feedback loops through which biology, social processes, and the environment cumulatively interact with each other in complex, inseparable, and unpredictable ways.

The Plastic Body

If the materiality of the body—its weightiness—could drag on the aspirations and desires of women with PCOS, what of changing this materiality through the new possibilities opened up by medical technology? The shifts in healthcare that I detailed in the earlier chapter have brought greater access to medical technologies, the medicalization of new avenues of life, and a greater emphasis on future quality of life. They have also meant greater possibilities for bodily alteration—whether cosmetic, through diet and exercise, or through reproductive medicine—to bring embodied experience more in line with women's desires, self-images, and interior subjectivities. Whereas it would be possible for women to focus on adjusting their desires or self-images such that they can be accommodated by their PCOS, my fieldwork suggested that, instead, interlocutors relied on interventions at the site of the body—or the fantasy of such interventions—to accommodate their desires and alleviate their distress. In doing so, they were treating the body as plastic and as an object to be molded to suit their aspirations.

At the least intrusive level, women with PCOS can recruit the technologies of nutrition and fitness in their body projects and body work. The dramatic rise in type II diabetes, cardiovascular disease, and other obesity-related lifestyle disorders in India, along with the move to slimmer body ideals and the increased acceptance of beauty work, has led to the emergence of a thriving diet and fitness industry (Bharathi and Dinesh 2018; Runkle 2003). Specialists and centers offering consultations, advice, and products have been especially concentrated in urban areas, and women of the urban professional middle class can access these quite easily, in terms of geography as well as economics. These goods and services hold the potential to not only reduce long-term health risks associated with PCOS, such as those of type II diabetes and heart disease, but they also offer women the possibility of altering their bodies to be more in line with lean body ideals.

Not many of my interlocutors had consulted personal trainers or fitness instructors. Instead, they relied on daily walks, yoga, dancing, or sporadic visits to the gym for exercise. The bulk of their efforts revolved around losing weight through dietary modifications; most of my interlocutors who had issues with PCOS-related overweight had consulted a dietitian or nutritionist at one point or another. Sometimes, this was on their own initiative; at others, it was the result of advice from their doctors. Regardless, most of them spoke of finding it very difficult to follow the prescribed dietary regimen. As I have described in Chapter 3 and Chapter 4, the social and expressive nature of meals in India, the cultural connotations surrounding food, and medical advice that targeted individuals rather than households presented barriers to their dietary management of PCOS. Life events that disrupted routines or made demands on women's time, attention, and energy resulted in the dietary management of PCOS being halted or abandoned. Such life events included changing jobs, stressful phases at work, marriage and a subsequent move to a different household,[1] weddings in the family, or childbirth. As they dealt with these disruptions, interlocutors ended up cycling through phases of watching what they ate and losing weight and periods of less restrained eating that led to weight gain.

However, for some interlocutors, the PCOS-related need to manage their diet and physical activity levels became part of their identities. Thus 29-year-old Mansi described how her PCOS had led to a career as a nutritionist. Diagnosed with PCOS as an overweight teenager, Mansi had been asked to lose weight to restore regular menstruation. Realizing that managing her weight would be a lifelong concern, she became increasingly interested in fitness and dietetics. She ended up specializing in clinical nutrition and the dietary management of medical conditions. Interestingly, she found that her professional identity as a nutritionist reduced barriers to the dietary management of her PCOS. For example, she explained about living with her parents-in-law:

> Actually, what happens is that now they just, they know that "You are a nutritionist, so that's how you're not going to eat [certain foods]". They understood that that way. So nobody tells me much nowadays. They're like, "You're a nutritionist, so whatever."

Thirty-one-year-old fitness instructor Bhakti had also found her career thanks to PCOS. Her bid to control her weight led to an interest in and commitment to exercise, as she left her job in business process outsourcing and opened up various fitness-related franchises.

Meanwhile, for 35-year-old Pooja, PCOS-associated weight gain led her to high-intensity CrossFit workouts that ended up becoming a passion. Pooja had a demanding career in finance, but she still woke up early to complete two hours of grueling training prior to starting the work day. Pooja told me that she loved the strength and power she could feel from her chiseled, muscular body. As she got more involved in CrossFit, she had shifted to a low-carbohydrate diet and had drastically cut her alcohol consumption; at one time, she told me, she would have found such abstention unimaginable. Here, it is important to point out that Pooja's household unit only consisted of herself and her husband. It was therefore easier for her to set her own schedule and dietary patterns. Nevertheless, for her, as for Bhakti and Mansi, nutrition and fitness technologies were important to an embodied sense of self and to their identities.

Besides diet- and exercise-related lifestyle changes, PCOS symptoms could be handled with medication or medical technologies. In terms of the cosmetic—hair and skin—aspects, topical treatments, oral contraceptives, or prescription isotretinoin could target acne issues and laser hair removal could help address hirsutism. Interlocutors did rely upon topical prescription drugs to treat their acne; such drugs were typically peeling and cell-communicating agents (such as salicylic acid, benzoyl peroxide, or tretinoin) or antibacterial creams. As these creams were externally applied, my interlocutors did not express misgivings about using them, and all my interlocutors with acne had used some form of such topical acne treatments.

Sometimes, these treatments could not completely clear their acne. In those cases, women would be prescribed oral contraceptives, or, in a couple of cases, the high-risk anti-acne drug isotretinoin. Prescriptions of these drugs met with far more resistance. Interlocutors spoke of wanting to "avoid medicines" or of their fears of "side effects" from "taking hormones [oral contraceptives]." Shruti, the public relations professional, remarked about her medication:

> I was on some combination of hormones and steroids. That meant mood swings, depression, irrational behavior—screwed up my marriage ... it is not part of your personality, it is actually the hormones you're eating.

Shruti stopped the medication as a result of these mood swings. However, the side effects that interlocutors referenced went beyond mood alterations, and women were worried about long-term effects on general health. As a result, interlocutors reported taking oral contraceptives at most for a few menstrual cycles, usually between three and six months. Not a single one of my interlocutors with PCOS had been or was on oral contraceptives long term, neither as a form of birth control nor as a means of managing her acne or regulating her menstrual symptoms (see also Chapter 4).

The case of Divya is revealing here. A 26-year-old working in marketing, Divya had been taking the drug isotretinoin despite vehement opposition from her family. Isotretinoin carries with it risks of fragile skin, joint pain and other musculoskeletal issues, mood disorders, blood cell issues, and compromised immunity. As a result, there are heavy prescribing restrictions on the drug. I asked Divya if she was taking isotretinoin because of the focus on image that came with her marketing job, but she replied that she felt "conscious for myself." Prior to taking isotretinoin, Divya had been prescribed an oral contraceptive, but a lack of any substantial changes to her acne, combined with a fear of long-term side effects, led her to discontinue the medication. Still, she took on the far more serious risks of isotretinoin in a bid to address her acne; she deemed the acne distressing enough to warrant such action. This was a common theme: the more the distress women experienced as a result of their symptoms and the higher the mismatch between their identities and the material realities of their bodies, the higher the degree of invasiveness and subjective risk they were likely to tolerate from their treatments. Furthermore, the greater the severity of symptoms, the more the attention and worry those symptoms commanded. As in Divya's case, even significant risks or highly invasive interventions were deemed acceptable for certain greatly troubling symptoms while being thought of as unacceptable for others.

When it came to hirsutism, all interlocutors with the symptom, that is, all hirsute interlocutors, had undergone or were undergoing laser hair removal sessions. Some went in for full-body treatments, whereas others, like Neha, focused on facial hair, which leads to the most gender confusion. Only Sunita, whose hirsutism—although present—was not very severe, said she chose not to undergo laser treatments because she found them too "drastic." Notably, although Sunita eschewed laser hair removal, she had relied on fertility treatments very early in her bid to conceive, as she had not been willing to wait to get pregnant.

Sunita was not alone in this. Four of my ten interlocutors with children had relied on ovulation inducers or fertility treatments to conceive (none, though, had undergone IVF). Biomedicine was here the preferred—indeed, the only—medical system drawn upon,[2] and biomedical reproductive technology represented freedom from doubt, waiting, and delays in conception. For example, Avni described being frustrated with one of her gynecologists who took a conservative approach, preferring her next doctor's more aggressive methods:

> [The new gynecologist was a] Sea-change from my [old] doctor. That was the first thing I noticed. She was younger, she understood my problems, like you know, she understood the problems of a couple who are both working. The problem was the frequency of making love was so less and then to have [sexual intercourse] on specific days, then there was travel, husband is traveling, I'm traveling, both of us are working throughout the day, you're tired, you don't have energy, you know? So she was very, very [clicks fingers] this with it—she was quite modern in her approach. She said, "*Yeh sab ho gaya, tumhara yeh* days *ways woh sab* [all this is done, your days (that fall within the peak fertile period), all that]. We're not doing this. We're going for IUI [intrauterine insemination]." That was the first thing she told me. Then she explained to me, what is IUI, and she said "I'll give you some injections and I'll give you some medicines to make you little bit—your egg—more fertile and accepting of the thing—and then we'll do an IUI." And I just blindly trusted her. I did not question her at all. I just like, me and my husband went together, we felt very comfortable with her, we connected with her because she could understand our problems.

Avni ended up conceiving within the first cycle of the IUIs, and she was so happy with the speed and results that she decided to rely on IUIs for a second pregnancy as well.

Not all interlocutors, however, were as happy with these technologies. Once they decided they would like to get pregnant, Sunita and Jaya initially chose to undergo fertility treatments rather than prolong conception in a bid to get pregnant without the aid of medical technology. A few cycles in, however, they discontinued treatments because of the way those treatments made them feel. Jaya, at 30, suffered an early miscarriage during her first cycle of fertility treatments. Shaken by this, she "decided to give her body a chance," stopped the treatments, and focused on increasing her levels of physical activity and on eating regular, balanced, and less calorie-dense meals. Within three months of making these dietary and activity-related lifestyle interventions, she conceived.

Sunita realized that she could not rely on the treatments alone. The preoccupation with getting pregnant was causing her too much stress, and her treatments were resulting in mood swings. "After doing two cycles," she recounted, "I decided to take a break because I thought I cannot do these cycles if I am going to get emotionally completely fried over it." She took a break from ovulation inducers and focused on losing weight. After she had lost 10 kilograms, she went back on ovulation inducers. "I thought," she explained, "I can't do this try [her luck, unaided by reproductive technology] and all." In her first cycle after the break, she conceived successfully.

Meanwhile, Fatima could not conceive after a few years of getting married, and, on her doctor's advice, started IUIs. After several unsuccessful cycles, she was frustrated, exhausted, and disappointed, and she wanted to get away from all doctors and medical interventions. Her husband thought they should start IVF, but after some discussion, they agreed to take a six-month break from all reproductive treatments instead. Ultimately, Fatima ended up conceiving during that time off.

The experiences of Jaya, Sunita, and Fatima underscore how the realities of assisted reproductive technologies are often frustrating, stressful, and time intensive. Nonetheless, interlocutors who were not immediately planning pregnancies spoke easily of the possibility of relying on these technologies. Reproductive technologies brought with them the option to delay childbearing until interlocutors felt they were ready for parenthood, and they allowed women to defer decisions about motherhood while keeping their options to have children open. My interlocutors spoke of their reproductive options as a spectrum that included fertility treatments, IVF, and, finally, adoption as the last stage.[3] Vidya, for example, told me, "I've always in my life wanted to adopt, so if this is it, if this is what it's going to take, I'll be very happy!" Priyanka said, about the possibility of infertility related to PCOS, "I thought worst to worst, we're not able to have a baby, we can always adopt." Niyati said that for both her and her husband, "adoption is always an option." Sucheta similarly told prospective grooms that she met through arranged marriage channels that because of her PCOS-related subfertility, "We'll try our level best to make it happen [through assisted reproductive technologies], but if it still doesn't happen, you should be ready for adoption."

A few points are worth highlighting here. First, as women from the professional middle-class segment, my interlocutors possessed the economic means to be able to engage with reproductive technologies and to even imagine doing so. India does not have a robust system of nationalized healthcare, and fertility treatments are not cheap. At the time of my fieldwork, non-IVF fertility treatments cost around INR 3,000–4,000 per cycle (approx. USD 40–50). Several cycles of these treatments, multiple diagnostic tests such as sonographies, and frequent consultations with doctors are typical in the journey toward successful conception. Furthermore, treatments are often preceded by intensive laboratory investigations to exclude male infertility factors or other issues. IVF is far more expensive; at the time of my fieldwork, it cost around INR 150,000 (approx. USD 2,000) per cycle.

Second, my interlocutors with PCOS had the sociocultural resources to contemplate relying on reproductive technologies. They knew about these technologies and could be proactive in seeking healthcare. Furthermore, as I discuss in the next chapter, the professional middle-class segment draws upon gender and conjugal norms and a closer engagement with modernity as a source of distinction. This allows for fertility and reproduction to become a concern only as couples start trying to conceive.

Third, reproductive technologies are often invasive and time consuming, they bring mood alterations and other side effects, require several attempts, and, in the case of IVF, have only modest rates of success. Nevertheless, women spoke of them as possibilities for the future without referencing these dimensions. The experiences of my interlocutors who went through these treatments showed that the reality of these treatments was far less attractive than their potential.

Fourth, the ease with which interlocutors spoke of the possibility of subfertility and of having to rely on reproductive technologies was noteworthy, given the rich literature on India that details the politics of silence and invisibility around reproductive health and reproductive failures (e.g., Bharadwaj 2016; Singh 2020; Unnithan 2019). The references interlocutors made to adoption are also significant. Aditya Bharadwaj (2003) has written about the cultural complexities surrounding infertility in India, such that "adoption is not an option." Yet, my interlocutors repeatedly mentioned adoption; this discrepancy is worth investigating further. Bharadwaj's study included members of the urban professional middle-class segment, which suggests that the easy comments of adoption as an option were not a class-based phenomenon alone. It is possible that women from this class segment saw adoption as far less of a threat than men—Bharadwaj could not always interview women separately from men—or that the intervening decade between his research and mine had seen a shift in attitudes. It is also very likely that with adoption, as with assisted reproductive technologies—or, indeed, infertility—the reality is far less acceptable than the possibility.

Medical Technology and Medicalized Possibilities

Drawing from Foucault's work on how dominant discourses are tied to disciplinary practices at the site of the body, Susan Bordo (1993), in *Unbearable Weight: Feminism, Western Culture, and the Body*, examined the production of feminine bodies. Bordo argued that women discipline their bodies through acts such as cosmetic surgery, dieting, hair straightening, makeup, and even exercise to produce appropriately gendered bodies that correspond to prevailing norms. These acts of disciplining are not just to avoid social sanction but also to gain a sense of control and pleasure. They are therefore often expressed as acts of creative expression or agency, and the structural forces that shape the experience of pleasure or pain in conforming to these to prevailing gendered norms go unacknowledged.

My interlocutors too represented their practices of laser hair removal, acne treatments, and diet and exercise as acts of self-care, undertaken so that they could feel better in their bodies rather than for socially instrumental purposes or as a result of oppressive expectations placed upon women. Even as they recognized the high economic costs of these technologies, they spoke of their availability, particularly of those services that medicalized cosmetic aspects (such as laser and acne treatments), favorably, for providing relief from the unhappiness caused by their symptoms. Nevertheless, the heightened focus on appearance in post-liberalization India and the ethic of "maximization of lifestyle" have been propelled and accelerated by the availability of these technologies. Although these technologies can help alleviate or mitigate symptom-related distress, they are implicated in exacerbating the sociocultural context that gives rise to such distress in the first place. On the other hand, lumping in technologies of nutrition and fitness with these other appearance-related disciplinary practices threatens to reduce them to being about presentability—the burden of which falls more heavily on women than men—alone. For Bhakti, Pooja, and Mansi, although their commitment to nutrition and fitness may have been motivated in part by appearance-related concerns, it was also about embodied wellness and the feeling of inhabiting a resilient, strong body.

The matter of assisted reproductive technologies is equally complex. Feminist scholarship has tended to look upon women's experiences of biomedicine, particularly reproductive technologies and the medicalization of childbirth, as disempowering (e.g., Bell and Figert 2010; Jordan 1993; Millard 1990; Padamsee 2011; Sandelowski 1991).[4] Reproductive technologies have been criticized for requiring women to endure high levels of risk, surveillance, and medication and for being promoted at the expense of allowing more time for conception and other lower-tech solutions. Moreover, they are implicated in rendering adoption and childlessness less socially acceptable. They deflect attention and resources away from environmental causes of subfertility to locate the problem—and its invasive solution—in individuals, usually women, instead. Linda Singer (1989) has argued in addition that such reproductive technologies, by allowing typically upper-middle-class women to delay pregnancy for careers, enable neoliberal regimes to mobilize women's bodies in the domain of production while still consolidating class privilege. Although early feminist critiques recognized that women could find these technologies empowering, they argued that they were also disciplining techniques that entrenched women's identities even more firmly in motherhood (e.g., Corea 1985).

As described, my interlocutors did speak of these technologies as liberating, and these technologies did allow them, as economically privileged women, to delay childbearing without worrying much about their fertility. Women could also opt for these technologies rather than trying to conceive without medical assistance; unassisted conception was a viable possibility even though it might have taken longer than assisted conception. In addition, as my interlocutors' experiences show, reproductive technologies were neither a guarantee of speed nor as easy and straightforward as they were perceived to be.

My interlocutors' experiences of the potential that these technologies represented cannot be dismissed. Frank van Balen and Marcia Inhorn have pointed out that much of the feminist literature criticizing reproductive technologies is "highly speculative, polemical, and even somewhat dismissive of an individual's legitimate reproductive desires and experiences" (2002: 6). Such literature, they argue, has typically been located in Euro-America, ignoring women in the Global South, and has often been more philosophical than empirical in its orientation. Indeed, Henrike Donner (2003) has described how, given the complex social relations surrounding childbirth and patrilocality in India, middle-class women in Calcutta experienced the biomedicalization of reproduction through caesarean sections as distinctly empowering.

For my interlocutors who engaged with reproductive technologies, this was a matter of their own choosing rather than one imposed upon them by their physicians; the choice to suspend that engagement was also very clearly theirs. These women were not submissive patients overwhelmed by biomedical authority. They regularly changed doctors, looking for those whose manner, approach, and advice suited them, and they challenged doctors' directives to take certain medications such as hormonal contraceptives or insulin sensitizers. They also stopped and started medication without supervision (see Chapter 4). For other interlocutors who did not actively engage with reproductive technologies, it was the *possibilities* that these technologies represented that were experienced as liberating. New reproductive options allowed interlocutors to feel a hypothetical sense of control over their future, such that they did not have to deal with the prospect of subfertility until they were ready to start a family. In this, they were aided by the new secular reasonings of risk and probability that I documented in Chapter 4. These new subjectivities oriented around risk meant that the consequences of PCOS could be thought of in terms of probabilities rather than as forces outside the realm of human negotiation. Imagining the future in medicalized terms granted women a sense of control over their circumstances. It allowed women to envision lives for themselves that were not immediately focused on childbirth, and it gave them the space to construct identities that did not revolve around the domestic sphere alone. Rather than linking womanhood to motherhood, in practice these technologies enabled the decoupling of the two (a theme I explore in more detail in the next chapter).

Embodied Subjectivities and Lived Experiences of PCOS

In Chapter 3, I referenced Margaret Lock's work on local biologies, which has challenged both the universal body that is common in biomedical models and the disembodied body of social constructionism. Lock's conceptualization of the body highlights instead the continuous, cumulative interactions between the biological and the social (Lock 1993; Lock and Kaufert 2001; Lock and Nguyen 2010). Local biologies linked to the "thin–fat" tendency among Indians are implicated in PCOS. Additionally, they play a role in which dimensions of PCOS draw attention and invite suffering for women.

Lock emphasizes that sociocultural differences do not just affect the body through epigenetics, diet, lifestyle, and environmental triggers, among other things, but that they are also significant in determining what dimensions of embodied experience, including of disease and bodily disruption, become foci of attention. Symptoms are socioculturally patterned, in that they represent features of bodily experience that are deemed significant enough within specific sociocultural worlds to warrant notice. Her observations find an echo in phenomenological assertions that our limited sensory and cognitive capacities mean that we are unable to experience the world in its entirety. Our consciousness is always directed toward certain aspects of experience, and other aspects, which do not receive our attention, recede into the background (Desjarlais and Throop 2011).

In listening to my interlocutors' narratives, I found that their attention to and concern regarding the symptoms they experienced and the health risks they faced formed a limited resource. These limited resources of attention interacted with assessments of significance at various life stages. Certain symptoms and concerns were centered at certain times while others became less immediate, shaping embodied experiences of the condition across the life course. Thus, presentability—once a concern only around the time when a woman was of marriageable age—had become an affective focus for women throughout their life course. On the other hand, fertility—which used to preoccupy women throughout their reproductive years—only came to the forefront as a concern once women started trying to conceive. Future health risks, when uncoupled from weight- and appearance-related distress, were the least noticed of all other dimensions of PCOS, and action to mitigate them rarely went beyond consumption-oriented token harm reduction practices.

For women of the urban professional middle-class segment in contemporary India, the changing sociocultural and technological landscape of the country had resulted in certain aspects of living with PCOS, such as those related to presentability, being foregrounded in experience while others, related to subfertility, had become less immediate. This dynamic, which dictated how much attention was devoted to dimensions of the lived experience of PCOS, was not static though. Limited resources of attention interacted with temporal factors and sociocultural contexts to influence where attention was directed at various life phases. This, in turn, affected local embodied experiences of PCOS. At any given point in time, the symptoms that received the greatest degree of attention also elicited greater degrees of distress or concern. These varying degrees of distress could be seen to explain women's changing levels of motivation when it came to implementing the diet and exercise-related interventions that were recommended in the management of PCOS. As medical practitioners noted in Chapter 4, commitment to lifestyle modification tended to peak around the life events of marriage and conception. In this chapter, I have highlighted, through my interlocutors' accounts, how technological advances affect subjectivities and sociocultural norms, which in turn influence the lived experiences of diseases, bodily disruptions, and health disorders. In the next chapter, I use PCOS as a window to examine shifting intimate modernities among the urban professional middle-class segment in greater detail.

Notes

1 In India, it is extremely rare for couples to live together prior to marriage; marriage therefore often implies a shift in residence. This shift can also (though not necessarily) mean a move to a patrilocal supplemented nuclear household of living with the husband and his parents. Larger joint family living tends to be much less common among the urban professional middle-class segment.
2 Alternative medicine is generally seen as better suited to chronic conditions and general wellness than to acute conditions or situations requiring quick results; see Chapter 4.
3 Interestingly, none of my interlocutors mentioned surrogacy, even though they mentioned IVF and adoption.
4 Much of this work privileges a putative "nature," setting up an opposition between the natural and the cultural/biomedical. Scholars such as Donna Haraway (1991) have contested this dichotomy, urging the use of new technologies for feminist ends.

6

"KIDS WILL BE A BONUS"

PCOS and Intimate Modernities

Despite the Indian government's decades-long focus on fertility regulation and family planning, India remains a largely pro-natalist society. Marriage and parenthood are critically important to a sense of identity, selfhood, and adulthood for both women and men. Additionally, marriage is a key rite of passage across castes, communities, and religions, and it is central to achieving mature gender status. Social sanction for childlessness and never-married status is extremely unusual and only granted for select roles that are associated with the periphery of the social order (such as those of ascetics, priests, or religious wanderers). Research on choosing to remain never married in mainstream society in India is virtually nonexistent, as such a choice is exceedingly rare and seldom voluntary.

For women, motherhood is viewed as part of a natural progression that follows after a few years of marriage (e.g., Mehta and Kapadia 2008; Riessman 2000). Although men are also expected to marry and have children, women disproportionately bear the burden of responsibility for both. Women are generally held accountable for reproduction and blamed for a couple's childlessness, and relatives tend to be more sympathetic to the men in childless couples than the women (Dhaliwal, Khera, and Dhall 1991; Jejeebhoy 1998; Mehta and Kapadia 2008; Mulgaonkar 2001; Singh, Dhaliwal, and Kaur 1997; Unisa 1999). Furthermore, childless women often face social isolation, accusations of inauspiciousness, ill treatment from affines, and marital abandonment. Unsurprisingly, given these conditions, anxiety, depression, and low self-esteem are widespread among childless women (Desai et al. 1992; Gupta 2000; Jeffery, Jeffery, and Lyon 1989; Jindal and Gupta 1989; Mulgaonkar 2001; Riessman 2000; Unisa 1999). Voluntary childlessness is exceptional, and in her study of childlessness in South India, Catherine Riessman (2000) found that even the few women she met who had chosen to be childless struggled with self-definition in the midst of their pro-natalist environment.

Celia Kitzinger and Jo Willmott's (2002) sociological study among women with PCOS in the United Kingdom found that through its effects on menstruation, appearance, and fertility, PCOS challenged women's perceptions of themselves as feminine. In India, given the emphasis on marriage and fertility, PCOS has the potential to similarly disrupt a woman's sense of

DOI: 10.4324/9781003171423-6

gendered self and to affect her matrimonial prospects, conjugal relationships, and life trajectory. As described in Chapter 4, healthcare practitioners
involved in the diagnosis and management of PCOS highlight subfertility as
one of its major features while simultaneously informing patients of the
potential to address fertility-related issues through medical intervention.
Most women with the syndrome successfully conceive, with or without
medical assistance, and women who are diagnosed with PCOS are informed
by their healthcare practitioners that subfertility need not imply childlessness. When it comes to PCOS, then, questions regarding fertility potential
are shrouded in uncertainty, opening up spaces for negotiations involving
reproductive desires, reproductive careers, and notions of appropriate family size. How do urban professional middle-class women with PCOS negotiate this uncertainty in India, and how does living with PCOS affect the
realization of women's identities within their conjugal relationships, their
experiences of intimacy with their husbands, and their life projects as linked
to family ideals? These questions form the focus of this chapter.

"It Doesn't Really Bother You"

Among women of the urban professional middle-class segment, PCOS did
not seem to carry any stigma, despite its connections to subfertility. My
interlocutors with PCOS viewed it as a condition that was part and parcel
of modern urban middle-class living, and they regularly mentioned that
they had heard, read, or been told by their doctors that around one in four
urban Indian women had the syndrome. Interlocutors said that they did not
feel embarrassed by the condition, and they spoke of openly talking about
and discussing their PCOS, even with men. For example, Vidya, the 29-year-
old marketing manager introduced in the earlier chapter, commented,

> I have no reservations about talking to anybody about [her PCOS].
> I mean this happened at work [having to rush to the doctor for
> menstrual issues], and my boss is a man. I mean I just told him
> I have to see the doctor ... I went back to work at about 8/8.15
> [pm], so he was still there, and he was like "What happened?" So
> I had to explain that I started bleeding, and it's okay. So he knows
> I have PCOS.

This was a common response; when I brought up the possibility that PCOS
might be something that women would wish to keep hidden, my interlocutors were surprised. Whereas it is possible that this openness reflected the
sample of my study, such that the only women willing to be participants
were those who were comfortable with having and talking about PCOS,
I do not believe this to be the case. For one, my interlocutors included
women who had endured a great deal of distress as a result of their PCOS,
with experiences encompassing reproductive issues, miscarriages, severe

hirsutism, and morbid obesity. Despite this, they seemed to have no hesitations in talking openly about the syndrome and their experiences of it. More importantly, however, my interlocutors' comments were borne out by my observations: PCOS was indeed spoken about easily and openly in this class segment, even in mixed company. Although the condition did not always come up in casual conversation, when it did, women admitted to a diagnosis despite being in the presence of family, friends, colleagues, or partners. I even contacted a few women with PCOS to be participants in my study through the recommendations of their male friends who heard about my interest in the syndrome. The ubiquity of the condition among the urban professional middle class undoubtedly aided this candidness. As 32-year-old Sucheta put it, "I did realize it's very common, and [nearly] everybody has it, and it's okay to have it."

In Chapter 5, I described how never-married interlocutors were not much preoccupied with future fertility. For example, the engineer Priyanka had stated about possible infertility that "When you're 18 and 19, it doesn't really bother you," and 23-year-old advertising executive Shabina equated worrying about infertility at her age to taking "unnecessary stress." At this life stage, interlocutors were instead focused on pursuing educational qualifications and career aspirations. Vidya clarified that at 29—an age by which most Indian women are married or contemplating marriage—reproduction was "not even high on my list of priorities right now." She was not married, and she was neither dating someone nor looking for prospective grooms through arranged marriage channels. She was completely happy with this state of affairs:

> So work for me is not really work. It is a part of me, it's part of my identity, and I give it my all. So, it's either all or nothing, always…. Majorelle [the brand she worked for; a pseudonym] is as good as my baby. I am my own full-time job. I really don't have time for someone else!

Sucheta, from the Marwadi community in which women are typically married by the mid-20s, also talked of delaying marriage in pursuit of her career goals. In her early 20s, she had a Bachelor of Commerce degree, was working at an international accounting firm, and wanted to get the Certified Public Accountant (CPA) certification. Her father queried her choices but did not oppose them:

> A time came, when I was about 22, like my dad did mention that "Are you sure you want to pursue a further degree, because then you'll be 25, and finding a boy may be difficult." In our community, you know, generally boys are into business, they have just B. Comm degrees and all that, or sometimes they don't even have a degree. So my dad was worried…. I would say that at the time when my dad

let me do the job and everything—he was little more liberal than the others—I managed to convince him; today, people are getting more liberal. My dad would appear to be a step behind.

Sucheta sat for her CPA exams in the United States and got her certification, and by the time she started "looking for boys," she was 29. She knew that her age, along with her PCOS, might be implicated in fertility issues. At the time, however, she wasn't worried enough to forego her professional aspirations.

During fieldwork, I found that these attitudes to fertility did not necessarily translate beyond the professional middle-class segment. My observations among young never-married women with PCOS from less than comfortably middle-class circumstances, for example, were very different. When I visited healthcare practitioners and government hospitals whose patient bases included the lower middle and working classes or when I participated in free medical camps conducted in slum areas, I encountered teenagers or young adults who were diagnosed with PCOS. Their mothers were distraught upon hearing that PCOS was associated with menstrual issues and subfertility. The mothers would ask the practitioners delivering the diagnosis regarding managing the fertility-related aspects of the condition, and they turned to the practitioners—and even the visitor anthropologist who was revealed to have PCOS herself—for assurances that their daughters could have children (see also Chapter 4). The mothers' anxieties seemed to amplify the worries of their daughters, who then went on to ask at length for strategies to combat their subfertility. The medical practitioners that I interviewed also told me that such anxieties regarding fertility were common among the more conservative "business communities." By this, they meant small-business-owning families from the Gujarati or Marwadi communities that typically fall within the petit bourgeoisie segment of the Indian middle class.

Negotiating Subfertility

The openness in talking about PCOS and limited concern with fertility potential that my professional middle-class interlocutors displayed was accompanied by an insistence on disclosing PCOS and PCOS-related subfertility to intimate partners. All my interlocutors who had been diagnosed prior to getting married had discussed their condition and its implications with boyfriends or prospective husbands. The views of Neha, a 32-year-old working at an investment bank, were widely echoed:

Now, there is more openness between men and women. You should be open about it. It shows the person's maturity; you'll know that you are marrying the right person.

When I met Neha, she had been divorced for a few years; her first marriage had been a casualty of her then-husband's infidelity. She was also newly affianced. Her friends had set her up with a common friend whom they thought would suit her, and the relationship had progressed from there. She considered this relationship an arranged match, and explained that the dynamics were different from those of her earlier relationship, which had been a "love marriage."[1] The subject of her PCOS had come up organically in that prior relationship. Her ex-husband (who was then her boyfriend) had seen her between waxing sessions, so he knew about the hirsutism that PCOS brought. "He had no problems. He didn't even comment. He was not bothered by it," she said. She had also not used contraceptives throughout the three years that she had been married to her ex-husband. That fact, combined with the advice she received from her endocrinologist, made her fairly certain that she would not conceive without assistance. Therefore, in her next relationship, Neha made a point of talking about the condition and its potential consequences in terms of not just her appearance but also her fertility:

> This time, it's an arranged marriage. My husband-to-be is older by five years. In a love marriage, there is that comfort level. Arranged, it's a little different. You don't know the person. It's a new thing, and nobody wants to settle for anything less than best....
>
> Before I arrived at a decision [regarding agreeing to get married], when we were heading toward it getting confirmed, I told him that I had irregular menses, that I would not be able to conceive without help. He told me "I am marrying you for companionship. If we don't have children, that is fine with me; how I look at you won't change"....
>
> See I have acne on my back also, there is the hair—I wanted to tell him about the cosmetic things also. I get laser [hair removal treatments] for my facial hair, but I am very conscious about it. Sometimes, you can see it. I didn't want him to be uncomfortable asking about it. I wanted to show him. I told him, "I want you to see; I want you to see and touch it." So, I showed him, I made him put his hand here [on her belly, where she had thick bodily hair], and feel it. He was okay with it.

Both her ex-husband and her prospective husband had seen companionship as the primary purpose of marriage and, like her, were not concerned with subfertility.

Shabina's boyfriend also knew about her PCOS. They had been dating for a year and a half, and he was familiar with the medications she was taking to manage the condition. Moreover, Shabina had also spoken to her boyfriend about the subfertility associated with PCOS. He was unconcerned, as he wished to be childless:

> He doesn't want kids. He is okay with not having kids and all that. I told him, "One kid *toh chahiye* [is required]." Because our marriage, if we ever get married, after 5–6 years, whatever, our marriage is not going to be easy because it is a religion problem. He is Hindu; I'm a Muslim, so there's already that issue.

Sucheta, who had waited to receive a CPA certification before meeting potential spouses through arranged marriage channels, had been similarly candid. By the time she had started meeting potential spouses, she was 29. She had wanted to settle into marriage before trying to conceive; this had meant that she would be in her early 30s—with a lowered fertility not only because of her PCOS but also her age—by the time she would start planning a family. She therefore made it a point to talk to prospective grooms about the possibility of infertility:

> I had very promptly discussed with the guys that "Are you okay? You're not marrying me for this, right? Because this should not be the reason that can create a rift between us. It may happen that I am not able to conceive. And I haven't gotten it [fertility] checked. I don't want to get it checked. Tomorrow, if I want to, and it doesn't happen, you should have that respect between us. We'll try our level best to make it happen, but if it still doesn't happen, you should be ready for adoption." You know, I told them very clearly....
>
> My [now] husband *toh*, I spoke to him about it, that "I don't know, I'm scared, but my age is 29 today. Tomorrow, I'm going to be 30, and 31, when we try, what if it doesn't happen? What if you're at fault, or I'm at fault, or something doesn't happen? So are you ready to take that heavy thing on your head that 'Yeah, I can live with it'? Because, we are at a stage also where we might not want to try for 3–4 years. You may want to try for a year or two, and then you might choose to take a call, you know, take a call, whether we want it [a child] or not."

Sucheta went on to use the men's responses to gauge her compatibility with them:

> See, more than anything what mattered to me was that they [prospective grooms] should be educated. And they should be broad-minded. As long as you are broad-minded and you understand, that was my concern. Most of them appeared to be okay. They didn't say anything.

For some, disclosure also meant informing the prospective spouse's family. A year into dating, Priyanka and her then-boyfriend started seriously discussing marriage. Her then-boyfriend was an only child, and his parents' only source of grandchildren. She therefore asked him to let his parents know about her PCOS and possible reproductive issues. "It was important for me that we start off with everything in the open," she recounted. Priyanka was, however, a relative outlier; most interlocutors felt that family members need not be informed. In Neha's words, "The decision is between him and me. There is no need for them to be told."

Overall, the narratives of my interlocutors reveal that prior to trying to conceive, they were not much concerned about their subfertility. Furthermore, they were making a point of discussing the possibility of childlessness with intimate partners and prospective spouses, and these partners were echoing and usually amplifying their lack of concern regarding fertility. This phenomenon was in direct contrast to the extensively chronicled focus on the fertility of women in India. Anthropological literature on India documents how women are scrutinized throughout their reproductive lives, even as adolescents or young unmarried adults, to ascertain their fertility potential; even elite class status has not been found to offer protection from the stigma of infertility (Inhorn and Bharadwaj 2007). My interlocutors' experiences therefore suggested a major shift in attitudes toward fertility among the urban professional middle class. In Chapter 5, I described how access to new reproductive technologies can be seen to be implicated in this shift. New reproductive technologies brought the possibility for professional middle-class women to put off motherhood until they felt ready to be mothers. Such technologies offered this potential even in the face of a fertility, already diminished by PCOS, that was likely to decline further with age. The new range of reproductive options contributed to letting women imagine lives for themselves that were not centered on childbirth, and they enabled the construction of more career- or individual-centered identities. In this, they assisted in the decoupling of motherhood from womanhood for women of this class segment. Such a decoupling has also been significantly aided by the shifts in conjugal and gender norms that have been taking place in post-liberalization India. I describe these in the next section.

The Turn to Companionate Marriage

In the arranged marriage and patrilocal, patrilineal household system in India, the conjugal unit was considered subordinate to the larger family. Conjugal intimacy was not just secondary to the interests of wider family bonds, but it was also typically actively discouraged as being dangerous to family and household harmony. As Susan Wadley pointed out, "if a woman seeks favouritism through her husband, the unity of the family is threatened" (2002: 16). Married women were aware of the disruptive potential contained in the pair bond and of the possibility of using sexual intimacy as a means of influencing husbands, but their opportunities for conjugal intimacy were heavily circumscribed (Jacobson 1982; Raheja and Gold 1994). Educated wives, especially in urban areas, were sometimes able to challenge the containment of the pair bond, but this was atypical. In fact, higher education could therefore work against a woman's marital prospects (Seymour 1999). Romantic love, although celebrated in folklore, romantic literature, and in Bollywood movies and songs, was not considered essential to successful married life. Indeed, it was often viewed as antithetical to the long-term success and stability of a marriage because, as an unruly emotion, it compromised objectivity and overrode family and community concerns (Mody 2002; Pinto 2011; Sharangpani 2010).

This began to change significantly after the economic liberalization of India. As mentioned in Chapter 2, middle-class women now face more opportunities and options for building careers and pursuing higher education, and the public visibility of women has become a marker of the urban professional middle class. This in turn has affected the domain of marriage. The overall age of marriage in India is still quite low, but it is changing among the urban middle class, as women complete their degrees or work for a few years prior to getting married. This has also altered relations between women, their affinal kin, and the patrifocal family. For example, the degree of power and authority that mothers-in-law wield has been declining:

> The "sandwich generation," where the cohort of women inform-
> ants were between the ages of 50 and 70, bemoaned the changing
> domestic space in which they were now sandwiched between their
> domineering mothers-in-law and intolerant modern daughters-in-
> law. The changing world of women, replete with new domestic vio-
> lence laws and new notions of womanhood had left them neither
> here nor there. As one informant said to me, her "time never came."
> (Sharangpani 2010: 273)

Meanwhile, as described in Chapter 2, access to new consumer choices and global media messages after the economic liberalization of India opened up a whole host of imaginary worlds. Media representations began to revolve around an idealized urban middle class that was portrayed as cosmopolitan, globally mobile, and comfortable with consumption. These new media messages drew a correspondence between sexual desire and the desire for consumer goods, such that Purnima Mankekar observed in her study of commodity erotics: "In contrast to earlier television shows, the programs of the 1990s displayed an unprecedented fascination with intimate relationships—particularly marital, pre-marital, and extramarital relationships—and contained new and varied representations of erotics (explicit as well as implicit)" (Mankekar 2004: 418–419). The "new" middle-class woman idealized in the media was a consuming subject who was confident in expressing her sexual as well as consumer agency. Nevertheless, her desire had to be domesticated by connecting it to conjugal intimacy; that is, her sexuality could only be acceptably expressed within the marital relationship (e.g., John 1998). Furthermore, the eroticization of the conjugal couple was a class-based project. For example, in *Shoveling Smoke*, an ethnography of advertising in India at the turn of century, William Mazzarella (2003) highlighted that contraceptives were advertised to the middle class as representing an aesthetic sexual experience but framed as a means of fertility control for lower-income "others." Conjugal intimacy came to be a middle-class ideal. Novel formations such as the matrimonial website, by complicating the already murky binary of "love" and "arranged" marriage more thoroughly, further aided these representations.

The terms "love marriage" or "arranged marriage" have always encompassed a confusing variety of matrimonial matches, and in contemporary India in particular, there need not be a clear set of differences between the two (Donner 2002). For example, candidates introduced to each other by their parents can still undergo a period of courtship similar to dating, whereas even individuals who have been dating tend to request parental approval for their union prior to getting married. The simplistic dichotomy of "love" or "arranged" marriage fails to recognize how these two categories are constantly produced and negotiated through familial performances. It also elides how kin recognition can provide social legitimation for marriages that were initially conceived as individual contracts rather than as social ones (Mody 2002). The love marriage vs. arranged marriage binary has also been critiqued for assigning individual agency only to love marriages and for ignoring nuances and overlaps between types of unions (e.g., Donner 2002; Kaur and Palriwala 2014; Uberoi 2008). For the middle class in contemporary India, a more companionate form of matrimony has become common even among so-called arranged marriages. This form accounts for the consent of the prospective bride and bridegroom and involves more private communication between them (Gilbertson 2014b; Fuller and Narasimhan 2008; Sharangpani 2010). Endogamous marriage is still the norm, but notions of companionate conjugality have become central to middle-class self-representations (Donner 2016).

My interactions in Mumbai suggested that whether a marriage was termed "love" or "arranged" was usually a product of the process through which the spouses were introduced to each other. A union resulting from the introduction of candidates through a matrimonial website was termed an arranged match, even when the prospective bride and groom had created their own profiles, shortlisted candidates themselves, and initiated contact. On the other hand, cases where a couple had met independently of such matrimonial channels (typically while at college, through work, or through common friends) and had been dating prior to marriage were termed love marriages, even when the formalization of the match had been contingent upon parental approval. Interlocutors also used terms such as "semi-arranged" to imply unions in which the woman had been approached by the prospective spouse, typically a man from within her community, with a view toward marriage that was provisional upon parental consent. Regardless of the terms used, I found that notions of choice were central to marital unions among the professional middle-class segment in Mumbai.

My interlocutors' narratives, whether those of married or unmarried women, revealed their expectations of companionate marriages. Women in relationships had spoken to their partners about their PCOS, and unmarried interlocutors used romantic partners' reactions to their condition to gauge compatibility and suitability for marriage. Indeed, Shruti, the PR professional mentioned in the earlier chapter, had divorced her husband because of his insensitivity when it came to her PCOS.

My married interlocutors' experiences also showed a new sense of priorities within marriage. Several spoke of their—and their husbands'—reluctance to subordinate conjugal intimacy to the pursuit of children. Sucheta told me of her husband's annoyance when her gynecologist advised them to schedule sex on particular days of her menstrual cycle, when chances of conception were highest:

> He's the type of person that he's clear that "I don't want to have a sexual relationship [just] because we want to have a kid." That really irritates him.

Niyati also mentioned resisting pressure from her doctor to conceive early to avoid reproductive failures. When she visited her gynecologist regarding her irregular periods prior to getting married, the gynecologist had advised her to plan early pregnancies. Once she was married—at age 25—the gynecologist suggested she try to conceive immediately and recommended that the newlywed couple schedule sex around Niyati's fertile periods to enhance chances of conception. However, Niyati and her husband had wanted a few years to settle into their marriage prior to embarking upon parenthood. When we spoke, Niyati was three years into married life. She and her husband still did not feel ready to be parents. Niyati spoke of her experiences with gynecologists and of an unwillingness to be rushed into pregnancy:

> Once, I visited after the wedding, he [the gynecologist] wanted to put me—he had given me a medicine which would increase my chances to get pregnant and had also suggested that on particular days of my cycle to try and conceive. Right after the marriage is what he suggested. But I was totally not up for it....
>
> Besides that doctor, I had gone to two other doctors for another opinion because my husband and I always wanted to know that is

this PCOD problem really a big factor for me to conceive. Because as far as both of us were concerned, we were not really prepared [to have children], and we didn't want to do it under a health pressure. Since I might not get to conceive later, since it might be more difficult later, we didn't want to try now—I mean, that was not the reason we wanted to try now. So, one of the doctors was like, okay, you want to wait for another year, but after a year, you should be trying. That has been their suggestion....

The kind of pressure that started coming in was a little frustrating, in terms of—when we got married—both my husband and I are like—he is two days older to me—so there wasn't much of an age gap. We got married when we were 25. At that point of time, the pressure to get pregnant was too much for him to deal with also. He was quite frustrated. But now, both of us are quite settled with it, that we're not doing this because of the health problem. If it has to happen, it'll happen.... We aren't looking at trying for another one and a half, two years. I'm 28 right now—so we're looking at trying only after about one and a half, two years, and we do realize that it will be a lot more difficult to conceive, but we—as of now—we've reached a decision where we'll see when we're prepared about it and we'll do whatever we can at that point of time. If it doesn't work out for us, for both of us adoption is always an option. So, it doesn't freak us out so much right now. We want to get pregnant for the right reasons, not because I may not conceive later.

Niyati and her husband realized that the likelihood of experiencing fertility issues increased the longer that they waited to conceive. Still, even when faced with the possibility of childlessness, they chose to focus on the conjugal aspects of their marriage rather than the reproductive dimension. Similarly, 30-year-old Anjali and her husband had decided early on that they didn't want to embark upon parenthood until at least five years into their marriage. Upon reaching that five-year mark, they had still not felt ready to be parents. They decided to wait for another two years, in spite of recognizing that the delay would be likely to affect their chances of conceiving.

Pragmatism, Reproduction, and Companionate Marriage

Even though interlocutors seemed not to be much bothered by subfertility prior to and early in their marriages, as chronicled in Chapter 5, PCOS-related subfertility came to the fore for many interlocutors as they began trying to conceive. Some interlocutors, such as Sucheta, who had brought up the possibility of childlessness or adoption with prospective spouses, described feeling distressed as childlessness began to seem more immediate and less abstract. A couple of interlocutors spoke of doubting their worth as wives. For example, 39-year-old doctor Renuka, a Catholic who had married her Hindu husband against both their families' wishes, recounted her time undergoing fertility treatments as highly taxing:

> When I got psychologically depressed was the sixth cycle [of ovulation inducers]. Fifth or sixth cycle I started going into depression, in the sense, doubt that it is not happening, not happening. Then ultimately I used to cry and tell my husband that, "I am not worth"—you know, "I cannot give you a baby." He was very supportive, he told me, "For me, you are important. I don't want this, we can even adopt a child"....
>
> For the first five months, having that intercourse, everything was okay. But then everything—it used to be religiously—ten days [planned sexual intercourse for the six to ten days around ovulation]—so I used to tell him, just do it so I can have a baby. Those kind of irritations I used to have. I used to be alone at home, *na*, after office hours, so I used to keep thinking, *ki* suppose my husband gets fed up, what is this, I am not able to give a baby. I prayed a lot. We did a lot of prayers. We went to temples, churches, everything. All that. This we started from the sixth cycle. Sixth cycle to the fifteenth cycle. "This cycle," she [the doctor] told me "is the last cycle. If this cycle is not successful, then we have to go to an IVF."

Ultimately, Renuka went on to have two children without relying on IVF.

Renuka's narrative reflects an ambivalence surrounding notions of marriage and reproduction that was not uncommon. Even as Shabina, 22 and never married, validated childlessness as an option for herself, she suggested that desire for children and womanhood went hand-in-hand: "See because, I'm a woman, at the end of the day, I would want a baby. I'm not saying I'm very modern, but yes, if I can't have a baby, that is also fine." Her statements reveal ambiguous and contradictory conceptualizations of the relationship between feminine identity and motherhood, and they expose the paradoxes that result from shifting gender norms.

Typically, this ambivalence only came to the fore as couples faced difficulties conceiving. Fatima, too, spoke of her feelings of insecurity as she underwent fertility treatments. Her husband Irfan, 11 years her senior, had fallen in love upon seeing her; he would go on to learn she was only 15 years old at that time. He waited until they could convince both their parents to approve the match, and they got married after she finished her bachelor's degree. When they married, she was 21, and he was 32. At five years into the marriage, they were still trying to conceive, and Fatima began to feel Irfan's age keenly. She worried that he had waited a long time to marry her only to have to wait again before they could have a child. She told him to divorce her and find another wife who could provide him with children; he assuaged her fears and told her to stop entertaining such thoughts. Ultimately, both Renuka and Fatima conceived successfully. Despite these positive outcomes, their experiences point to how subfertility becomes a matter of concern for women. Their descriptions highlight the persistence of the centrality of childbearing to normative feminine biographies, in spite of a shift toward companionate marriages.

Nonetheless, it is worth pointing out that all my interlocutors, even those trying to conceive or undergoing fertility treatments, demonstrated a new set of goals when it came to marriage. As Neha put it, "Priorities have changed. I would rather have a stable relationship than kids. Kids will be a bonus." Along with these changed priorities, some married interlocutors also expressed ambivalence toward or an outright rejection of parenthood. One interlocutor, for example, said, "I'm not sure I need kids in my life." Anjali, who had put off conception at six years into her marriage, was unequivocal, "It's a choice. I can live my life without a baby." Two other married interlocutors with PCOS, one aged 30 and the other 34, were open about their decision to be voluntarily childless. Given that motherhood has been a mandate for women in India, the fact that women were treating child-rearing as a choice is noteworthy. Much as the narratives of my professional middle-class interlocutors suggested comfort with childlessness and the embracing of new family ideals, as mentioned, the realities were more complicated.

Interlocutors' disclosure to intimate partners regarding their PCOS-related subfertility must therefore be considered against this complex backdrop and in relation to established marriage practices in India. Contemporary conventions of arranged marriage in India include the management of expectations regarding the future, especially in relation to household roles and responsibilities toward parents, relatives, and communities, among other things. Thus, the prospective spouses—and often their families—discuss or negotiate issues such as whether the woman will work outside the home after getting married, whether the household will be patrilocal or nuclear, broken engagements or divorces within families, smoking/drinking habits, dietary preferences and proscriptions, and so on (see also Lukose 2009: 125–128). Marriages have a greater chance of succeeding when expectations are clear, aligned, and acceptable. For women and their families, for whom the social consequences of unhappy or unsuccessful marriages are much heavier, such expectation setting is especially critical, and pragmatism toward negotiating lifestyle, economic, and future expectations has continued even after the turn to companionate marriages (Ahearn 2001; Osella 2012).

For my interlocutors, discussing their PCOS, its symptoms, and potential subfertility was part of this pragmatic negotiation of expectations as they contemplated or entered marriages. Such negotiation was aimed at managing the practical dimensions that are thought to contribute to long-term marital stability. This was regardless of whether those marriages were termed love, arranged, or semi-arranged. These negotiations, while creating space for women's individual aspirations, were also attentive to family and community concerns. They helped women mitigate the social consequences of their PCOS and to gauge the potential of their prospective alliances to lead to companionate unions.

"Supportive" Partners

By negotiating potential issues and setting expectations, interlocutors were also assessing how likely prospective spouses were to support their aspirations and wellbeing. Married interlocutors with PCOS overwhelmingly spoke of "supportive" husbands or of having their "husband's support." Unmarried women looked for supportiveness in their partners; candidates that were thought unlikely to be supportive were deemed to be unsuitable long-term prospects. Shruti, who spoke of her ex-husband as not having been supportive, had filed for a divorce as a result. Upon querying women on what being supportive in the context of PCOS entailed, I came to realize that it revolved around two major themes.

The first was managing the affective dimensions of living with PCOS. This included assuaging fears and alleviating distress resulting from symptoms (especially appearance- and reproduction-related ones), accompanying women to doctor's visits, and being a stable presence in the face of the mood alterations caused by the syndrome and medications to manage it. For example, Bhakti, who had met her husband through a matrimonial website, spoke of her husband's ability to deal with her hormonal ups and downs: "He's very good at that. He is very good. Initially, we used to have arguments, but once he realized, now, he becomes very calm.... He's taken it very calmly." When asked if he was generally a calm person, Bhakti laughed: "The only person he is calm with is me." Similarly, Shabina said of her boyfriend,

> So, he knows, about my periods and all. I need to get—he needs to get—through those seven fucking PMSing days, right? [laughs] So at that time I told him, this is PCOS, this is the scene. So, he's pretty cool with it; he'll tell me *ki* take care of yourself, and he'll take care—he himself wakes me up at 6 o'clock[2] and tells me "Go, bloody, go for yoga it's good for your PCOS."

Mumtaz, meanwhile, relied on Aamir to help her through the stresses and anxieties of the fertility treatments she was undergoing. She preferred talking to Aamir about these issues over talking to her mother:

> I basically speak to him, because he's, first of all, he is a very good friend of mine, and then he's my husband. So I always discuss whatever problem I have with him only. And he's like a very cool type of a person. Like "It's not working out; it's okay. Next, we'll do the next trial."

Fatima similarly spoke of the emotional steadiness of her husband, Irfan, who calmed her fears of childlessness and told her that he "was okay with kids or no kids."

The other major aspect of support involved protecting conjugal privacy by asserting boundaries with the larger family. Such drawing of boundaries mattered regardless of whether the couple was in a nuclear, supplemented-nuclear, or joint family. Childlessness is highly visible in India, and family members, friends, acquaintances, and even perfect strangers easily ask personal questions about family composition and plans. For women trying unsuccessfully to conceive, such questions are unwelcome and painful, and navigating them appropriately is socially complicated. Mumtaz, five years into her marriage and childless, could not keep her fertility treatments hidden from friends and family. This meant, though, that "since everybody is knowing that we are going through this treatment, people keep asking, 'How is it working out?' and all." She found the questions intrusive and had a hard time protecting her privacy without offending people. In such cases, her husband Aamir proved crucial to evading others' curiosity. "Now," she told me with a laugh, "Aamir takes over." When I spoke to Aamir, he explained,

> Lot of outsiders, like friends, or friend's friends, they are more interested, "*Kya ho gaya, kya ho gaya* [what happened, what happened?]". See for me, it doesn't matter. Because my nature is not that. I am more chill, more calm. But for her, it really affects her. You have to know where to draw the line. There are some people who are more interested, you know, "Why it's not happening?" blah blah blah. "It's been so long since you are married." These things are there. Plus, being from a Muslim family, people are more interested, outsiders.... It affects her a lot.... I have my own way of handling them. I tell them like, "It will happen; we'll give you the good news soon." Stuff like that. Just to change their focus. I'm more used to handling them.

Supportive husbands also recognized that women bore the brunt of the social scrutiny that resulted from fertility issues and childlessness. They therefore worked to shield wives from such social scrutiny. Farhan pointed out, for example, that "Being a girl, there's a lot of additional—I would say a lot of undue responsibility—that 'I have to fulfill the expectations of the family, I have to start the family'."

A husband's assistance with asserting boundaries was even more critical when it came to affinal kin. Archana, who had given birth to her daughter at age 34, told me, "They [in-laws] would have wanted to [tell us to have a child earlier], but our [her and her husband's] deal is, we are very clear about setting up boundaries, so they never overstepped that." Similarly,

35-year-old Avni, pregnant with her second child and living in a supplemented nuclear household with her parents-in-law, mentioned of her
husband,

> He conducts himself also like that.... Here, it's his show. The other
> people are—I mean they are there, but they are not the lead. That
> also establishes the—the soft things [lack of boundary crossing
> from family members].

As a result, she said, "I have never been told by relatives that 'Why have you
not conceived?'"

Women thus relied upon their husbands' supportiveness in their companionate marriages. My married interlocutors were usually accompanied to
gynecologist visits by their husbands, as opposed to by their mothers, sis-
ters-in-law, or mothers-in-law, and all my married interlocutors confided in
their husbands about PCOS-related concerns. Husbands were not just as
emotional allies but also vital in protecting conjugal privacy from intrusion
by outsiders, even when those outsiders were other members of the larger
family. Such spousal support is significant, as it was not the norm for middle-class women from an earlier generation (e.g., Liddle and Joshi 1986).

Fertility, Gender Norms, and Middle-Class Distinction Projects

Dimensions of not just generation, but also class, are worth highlighting
further here. As members of the urban professional middle class, my interlocutors had geographic, economic, and sociocultural access to reproductive technologies. Moreover, the ubiquity of these reproductive services and
the pervasiveness of the PCOS diagnosis among the urban professional
middle class have helped normalize both PCOS-related subfertility and a
reliance on fertility treatments for this class. The lived experiences of PCOS
among women from other socioeconomic strata, who may not possess similar resources, are likely to be very different. Class also played a role in terms
of the new ideals of companionate marriage and supportive partners that
further contributed to women's resilience in the face of subfertility.

As detailed in Chapter 2 and Chapter 3, in post-liberalization India,
increased opportunities for education and employment have come to define
the urban middle class. Among the professional middle-class segment,
women are also expected to show greater engagement with "the modern"
while still balancing their commitments to "tradition." Gender claims have
long been used by the middle class in India as markers of distinction. The
middle class locates itself in opposition to the "corrupt" West and
Westernized elite as well as the "uncivilized" lower classes through claims
that have typically revolved around norms for and expectations of women
(Deshpande 2003; Srivastava 2007). It is therefore interesting to find that

118

new claims of supportiveness from men, as referenced in my interlocutors' narratives, were also being drawn on as markers of distinction for this class.

In addition to gender norms, the middle class in India has also always drawn upon practices related to fertility and childbearing as part of a class-based identity project. The smaller family sizes of the middle class have been used to distance this class from the lower socioeconomic orders, which, with their high number of children, are portrayed as unruly, illiterate, and regressive (Béteille 1992; Donner 2006; Srinivas 1994). I argue that in post-liberalization India, limited concern with fertility is also part of the distinction project of the professional middle-class segment. In her study of narratives surrounding middle-class marriage in Sri Lanka, Asha Abeyasekera (2016) found that the contrast between representations of the "traditional" past and the "modern" present hinged on the idea of exercising choice regarding whom to marry rather than on notions of "love." My conversations in Mumbai revealed that it was similarly the idea of exercising choice in terms of whether and when to have children with supportive partners in companionate marriages, rather than the realities of voluntary childlessness, that marked middle-class self-representations.

Lay professional middle-class interlocutors constantly stressed that attitudes to childbearing had been changing among their class segment. For example, 38-year-old Shefali, who had adopted a child when she had been unable to conceive, observed,

> *Atta khoop* change *zhalay* [There has been a lot of change]. Everybody is changing; the generation is changing. Even mothers-in-law are working. There is no pressure—marriages are late. Marriage is happening at 28/29. They think of a family only in their 30s. *Purvi, barech* question marks *asayche* [Earlier, there would be a lot of questions if a woman could not conceive]. Last ten years there have been a lot of changes.

Echoing Shefali's perspective, a 38-year-old homemaker remarked that "'a child is the ultimate'—that mindset is changing," and a 31-year-old male interlocutor stated that when it came to life biographies and marriages, "these days kids is not the only thing."

Interlocutors were, however, careful to provide the caveat that these changed attitudes were not always reflected among other classes. Prashant, a 26-year-old engineer, told me of friends of his, a married couple, who had been facing fertility issues. They were both highly educated, Prashant made a point of telling me. This meant that they did not have to endure familial pressure to conceive; the husband's family "were okay with the woman having some problem." Their experience, he clarified, was not typical outside of educated and professional members of the urban middle class. "It depends upon the guy," he said, before elaborating, "I mean it depends upon the dynamics of how the guy and the girl work." He then went on to talk of the larger family context of couples as relevant. In communities that are dominated by "business families," he said, a "a girl can get rejected" by prospective spouses or affinal kin because of reproductive issues. Interlocutors thus felt that reproductive issues were more likely to result in negative social consequences in the past, in rural areas, among the working and non-middle classes, among "business" communities, and in cases where women were not very highly educated. They were therefore marking out the urban professional middle class as more gender progressive than other socioeconomic strata, and distinguishing it from rural populations, nonprofessional communities, the lesser educated, and past generations.

Whereas these statements reflect the new prerogative for urban professional middle-class women of not having to deal with fertility potential until they actively start trying to conceive, they also draw from entrenched discourses regarding family planning and the progressive, respectable middle-class family. Although population control has been a focus for the Indian state ever since the country gained independence in 1947, family planning policies have overwhelmingly targeted the poor. In population control and family planning discourses, the poor have been associated with a higher number of children, symbolizing a lack of modernity and general backwardness. In these discourses, it was "the responsible middle-class mother, who by practising birth control, proved herself to be educated and by extension capable to bring up the right kind of young citizen" (Donner 2006: 372). As noted before, the post-liberalization idealization of sexual desire bounded within the conjugal pair is also tied to this class framing. The relative lack of concern with fertility potential among the professional middle-class segment is another aspect of this class project.

PCOS, Class, and Intimate Modernities

Theorists of modernity have argued that the modern era is marked by distinctive changes in the domain of the intimate (Giddens 1992; Beck and Beck-Gernsheim 1995; Beck, Giddens, and Lash 1994). In particular, Anthony Giddens (1992) has theorized that late modernity brings a turn toward a sexuality unfettered from earlier imperatives of reproduction and toward egalitarian "pure" relationships that fuse sexuality with love. He also suggests that these changes in intimate relationships are aided and accompanied by increased individualism and reflexivity. This, Giddens argues, allows for life decisions that are made less as a matter of course and more after careful deliberation.

Although modernity is indeed accompanied by changes in the intimate dimensions of marriage, sexuality, and family life, those changes are rarely as homogenous and universalized as these models suggest. Ethnographic studies have shown that contrary to these dominant—but empirically thin—models, "intimate modernities" (Donner and Santos 2016: 1126) are heterogeneous, complex, and shaped by their local social and cultural contexts (e.g., Ahearn 2001; Donner 2002; Donner and Santos 2016; Friedman 2006; Hirsch and Wardlow 2006; Jamieson 1999; Mody 2002; Osella 2012; Osella and Osella 2006; Yan 2010). Most anthropological studies of intimate modernities in post-liberalization India have tended to revolve around love, conjugality, and companionate marriage. The relationship between those dimensions, "modern selves," and fertility and reproduction has, however, not received much attention. Studies of family projects, even in post-liberalization India, have been dominated by a focus on childlessness and the social consequences it brings.

My professional middle-class interlocutors exhibited a rather different relation to fertility than that chronicled by this literature. Their reproductive potential did not concern them much until they were ready for childbearing. Post-liberalization changes in India have destabilized older gender and conjugal norms, such that the automatic linking of femininity, fertility, and conjugality is being disrupted among the urban professional middle class. This class segment defines itself through the higher educational and professional qualifications of women. In addition, women of this class segment are expected to show greater engagement with the "modern" than women of previous generations and women from other segments of the middle and not-quite-middle classes. As a result, they have greater opportunities to explore aspirations and identities, such as professional ones, that were previously far less accessible.

As I mentioned in Chapter 3, the identity of housewife was not a desired one among my interlocutors. My interlocutors with PCOS defined themselves through their educational or career-related credentials (even those who were not working outside the home at the time of my fieldwork), and they did not see themselves as defined only through marriage, motherhood, or the private sphere. Their cultural capital allowed for emphasis to be taken off the realm of reproduction, and their economic capital enabled access to the new medical technologies that helped make subfertility less of an immediate concern. Together, this facilitated a wider range of life choices. Later marriages and the ubiquity of PCOS in this class segment have additionally meant that subfertility is much more common and therefore less a source of stigma. Meanwhile, companionate marriage ideals have placed companionship, rather than biological and social reproduction, at the heart of the institution of marriage; this further helped make fertility potential less of a concern. Women among this class segment privileged companionship over fertility and negotiated expectations regarding family size and marital priorities with their partners, whether they were in relationships deemed "arranged," "love," or something in between. They expected supportive partners, and those partners played crucial roles in mitigating the negative dimensions of possible reproductive failures. This was very much a class-based phenomenon.

Moreover, these attitudes were complicated by the realities of the distress caused by lived realities of subfertility as women started trying to conceive.

In the pro-natalist environment of India where motherhood is prized, marriage has been treated as a means toward motherhood, and women have been evaluated throughout their reproductive lives for their fertility potential, experiences of subfertility could leave women feeling profoundly insecure about their worth as wives. There was not so much a decoupling of conjugality from fertility as much as a representation of these two as separate domains of the intimate. It was, then, the treatment of childbearing as a choice that was central to professional middle-class self-representations and projects of distinction. While the narratives within this class segment suggest a greater focus on individual choice and identity, this focus does not in praxis displace broader normative structures of family life.

Furthermore, the shift toward a greater emphasis on choice and individual identity does not imply that social and familial ties hold no sway. Instead, they are navigated in novel ways. Thus, supportive partners are enlisted in negotiating the tricky terrain of protecting conjugal privacy without sacrificing ties to wider kin and social networks. Conjugal relationships also involve balancing individual and social desires through the negotiation of expectations with prospective partners and future affines prior to matrimony. These relationships are not quite the "pure" individual-oriented relationships that free sexuality from reproductive imperatives that have been predicted by the dominant models of the intimate in the modern era. The reality is rather more complex. Still, the turn toward companionate marriage, expectations of supportive partners, and access to new reproductive technologies have allowed women to be less concerned about their fertility potential, and this has contributed to women's resilience in the face of PCOS-related subfertility.

Notes

1 The boundaries between "love" and "arranged" marriage are murky and difficult to draw, as I elaborate upon further in this chapter. I have replicated Neha's use of the terms here.
2 This was over the phone. Shabina lived with her parents. Although she had told her mother about her boyfriend, her father did not know.

7

CONCLUSION
Toxic Disruptions

PCOS is seen—by women with the condition as well as by others in urban middle-class India—as a disorder of modernity. It is at once a symbol of the rapid and widespread political–economic, environmental, and socio-cultural changes that India has undergone in the last couple of decades and an embodied manifestation of the biosocial stresses and harms accompanying those changes. The structural burdens and accelerated environmental degradation and pollution implicated in vulnerability to PCOS correspond to shifts in political–economic structures following the liberalization of the Indian economy. A lay epidemiology of PCOS, in particular, highlights these shifts and blames them for a toxic relationship between the body and its environment that manifests in a general lack of wellness and a rise in chronic conditions and metabolic disorders (Chapter 2).

For women with the condition, however, PCOS is also a lived reality. The syndrome is a disruption in their lives. It can bring great distress, as it affects their embodied sense of self, their appearance, and their reproductive aspirations. It raises risks of future health complications related to metabolic syndrome issues such as those of type II diabetes and heart disease. Indians are already more vulnerable to these metabolic conditions as a result of the Indian "thin–fat" tendency to be metabolically obese even at morphologically slim body weights. The successful management of PCOS requires motivation and discipline in making lifestyle changes, competency and deftness in negotiating culturally patterned expectations regarding sociality, care, and gender roles, and significant cost outlays.

In the lives of urban professional middle-class Indian women, PCOS is a disruption linked to a toxic location. As detailed in Chapter 3, women from the urban professional middle class face several structural burdens throughout their life course, and these burdens start early and last well into middle age. The time around menarche (the start of menstruation)—a critical and vulnerable developmental time—is also the time when middle-class girls face numerous pressures. An unrelenting focus on exam preparation leads to drastically circumscribed physical activity, long days and sleep-deprived nights, and few avenues for leisure or play. Multiple stressors thus buffet the vulnerable young body, rendering it susceptible to PCOS. Stressors then

DOI: 10.4324/9781003171423-7

continue to pile up—in adolescence, as young women compete for limited educational positions; in their 20s, as women compete for career opportunities; and once married, as they bear the double burden of work within and outside the home and as they juggle multiple roles. These structural burdens placed on urban professional middle-class women interact with the "thin-fat" local biology and an urban environment rife with EDCs in ecosocial loops. Together, they not only render women highly vulnerable to PCOS but also pose barriers to the condition's successful management, exacerbate symptoms, and increase risks of associated metabolic health conditions. What does it mean and feel like to live within such a toxic location while managing the consequences, and what can those experiences tell us about post-liberalization India? These two questions have animated this book; I have investigated what it means to be a woman from the urban professional middle class living with PCOS in contemporary India, as well as how the condition and the experience of living with the condition can shed light upon wider changes occurring in middle-class life in the country.

Toxicity, Gender Nonconformity, and PCOS

There can be no denying that EDCs adversely affect ecologies, disrupting the health and reproductive capacities of living beings. Much of the popular concern with EDCs and their toxicity has centered on the "gender-bending" aspects of EDCs and the threats that they pose to "normal" human bodies. While pointing to the harms of EDCs, such discourse nevertheless risks deepening the marginalization of certain kinds of bodies that are portrayed as "abnormal," and it is often rooted in antiqueer heteronormativity. That is, such discourse plays into suggestions that there is a "correct" way to be male or female, such that any body not fitting that paradigm is categorized as abnormal. In addition, it ignores intersex realities and the inequalities that they bring. Feminist, trans, and environmental justice scholars have therefore tasked social scientific studies on toxicity with chronicling the health harms of EDCs—particularly their effects on reproduction—without marking certain bodies, especially gender nonconforming ones, as deviant or defective (Agard–Jones 2013; Ah-King and Hayward 2014; Cielemęcka and Åsberg 2019; Di Chiro 2010; Murphy 2017).

PCOS has adverse effects in terms of an idealized feminine appearance (acne, hirsutism, scalp hair fall, overweight) and reproductive potential. As such, it threatens women's abilities to fulfill conventional gendered norms and expectations. As described in Chapter 5 and Chapter 6, my interlocutors with PCOS drew upon medical technology to address the appearance and subfertility-related aspects of the condition. As women of the professional middle-class segment, they possessed the economic means and knowledge to engage with these technologies. These technologies were also geographically accessible to urban professional middle-class women by virtue of these women being in a well-served metropolis. By engaging with medical services to domesticate their unruly bodies into conforming with the ideal for a feminine appearance, especially in terms of hirsutism, which was perceived as worryingly gender-bending, women were implicated in that ideal becoming more firmly entrenched. In alleviating their personal discomfort, they were exacerbating the marginalization of others with non-conforming bodies who might not possess their resources.

The dimension of fertility was, however, more complicated. As noted in Chapter 6, women spoke of the possibility of relying on reproductive technologies to address their subfertility, and access to such technologies gave them the leeway to think of whether and when to bear children as a choice. In this, they were aided by emergent intimate modernities—new family ideals and conjugal norms—among the urban professional middle-class segment. Some of my interlocutors with PCOS could therefore express ambivalence toward or an outright rejection of childbearing and child-rearing. Against the backdrop of a country in which motherhood has been treated as a mandate for women, this was conspicuous and significant. Here, women affected by toxicity were challenging conventional heteronormativity and pro-natalism.

Fieldwork revealed that it was the behavior-related aspects of PCOS that were deemed gender disruptive that had the most potential to be used to further antiqueer and heteronormative commentary. This was most notable, for example, in the quotes of the two (perhaps unsurprisingly) older male homeopaths detailed in Chapter 4, who thought PCOS could be attributed to women behaving in "unfeminine" ways or to their not "accepting their femininity." This was, however, very much a minority view. The dermatologist Dr. Fernandes framed the typically higher testosterone[1] levels of women with PCOS in far more neutral terms. She saw these elevated testosterone levels as resulting from the multiple demands placed on the time and resources of women. For her, they were implicated in fueling the aggressiveness that enabled women to meet those complicated demands, even as they brought adverse effects on wellness and future health outcomes.

Women with PCOS themselves spoke of the possibility of their having higher testosterone levels than other women far more positively. For example, as described in Chapter 5, the neurobiologist Sunita suggested that women with PCOS—given that they had elevated testosterone levels—were likely to be more driven and therefore more suited to the new realities of a highly competitive workplace. She also wondered whether PCOS was in a way adaptive, giving women with the condition a selective advantage for their environment. Similarly, two other women with PCOS joked about being more driven and aggressive, which they represented as positive traits, as a result of their PCOS and higher androgen levels.

Two aspects are worth highlighting here. For one, it was not the gender nonconforming bodies of women with PCOS that were being deemed deviant by the homeopaths but rather their gender nonconforming *behavior*, which was in turn blamed for PCOS. As I have documented throughout this book, gender norms have been changing among the professional mid-dle-class segment toward more engagement with the "modern." Among this class segment, more conventional ideas regarding women's appropriate aspirations and behavior are being dismantled, and women are encouraged and expected to build identities related to education, employment, and consumption rather than the domestic sphere alone. The comments from the two homeopaths point to the fact that older notions of appropriate feminine behavior nevertheless persist, albeit as residues. New behaviors, unwelcome to some, were welcomed by others. The women with PCOS who regarded their aggression as a positive trait were speaking to the new gender norms that they espoused. In particular, they—and Dr. Fernandes—were referencing the increased and higher expectations, in terms of balancing multiple roles within and outside the home, placed upon women from this class segment. They were suggesting that PCOS enabled their fulfillment of those expectations. In this formulation, PCOS was not necessarily a negative state, and the exposure to toxicity, or intoxication, contributing to it was a useful intoxication. The condition—a result of women's position within a toxic location—became a biological feature that also helped them navigate that location more successfully.

The Intoxication of Toxic Locations

This acceptance, even valorizing, of PCOS points to the fact that toxicity and its health results need not always be feared or dreaded. Not all intoxication is unwilling or unwelcome; individuals can intentionally engage with toxic chemicals for the advantages they bring, whether these be improved productivity, skin lightening, wakefulness, or the opportunity to experiment with sexual identities (Hardon 2021; Pine 2016). Elizabeth F. S. Roberts (2015) has documented how lead-glazed ceramic dishes continue to be used by families in Mexico, despite the detrimental effects of lead being known, because they represent ties to the past, carry religious significance, or are thought to make food taste better. In another study, Roberts's (2017) interlocutors in a working-class neighborhood in Mexico City saw their toxic location, enclosed by freeway exhaust, cement dust, and a sewage-laden dam, as bringing much-desired stability and protection from disruptive police and public health surveillance. Despite their negative consequences, not just toxicants but also toxic locations can therefore be considered acceptable because of the advantages they are seen to bring, even by those exposed to them.

Toxic locations need not just be tolerated with forbearance; they can also be actively intoxicating. I use the term "intoxicating" here in the dual sense of allowing entry to toxicants as well as to reference the potential for heady and addictive effects. Even as my interlocutors acknowledged the harms of their toxic location—the stress, the reliance on quick fixes, and the pollution and environmental contamination—they nevertheless enjoyed the opportunities that such a location brought—the ability to claim identities related to being "modern" Indians, cosmopolitan consumers, urban professionals, and companionate partners. These identities—and thus these locations—carried pleasures. As described in the earlier chapters, urban professional middle-class women's subjectivities have been structured by the political–economic shifts of post-liberalization India, such that these identities were highly desired. An inability to engage with these identities brought pain, and women were not willing to forego the pleasures of these identities to preserve their health. Jacqueline's quote in Chapter 3 about not wishing to slow down, which caring for her health would require her to do, reflected much broader attitudes. Mitigating exposure to toxicity required interventions in terms of lifestyles, geography, socializing, and aspirations that women did not manage to make (see Chapter 5); the social and personal costs of these changes were judged to be too high.

Indeed, as an Indian woman from the professional middle-class segment with PCOS myself, when I wonder whether I would have liked to come of age and live in pre-liberalization India if it would spare me PCOS, the answer is an unequivocal "no." I too am a product of my time and my class and cannot imagine willingly giving up the pleasures of modernity, urban living, consumption, beauty work, financial independence, companionate relationships, childlessness, and employment outside the home that post-liberalization shifts have made more acceptable and much less of a social struggle. PCOS, given that it currently causes me little distress, seems a rather small price to pay. Like other Indian women with PCOS from the urban professional middle class, I am intoxicated by my lifestyle and aspirations and do not wish to renounce them.

Harm Reduction

Instead of renouncing their position at the interface of several ecosocial pressures—and the myriad pleasures that position offered—my interlocutors with PCOS focused on reducing its harms, whether biological or sociocultural. They harnessed medication and medical technology to manage their symptoms and augment their fertility (Chapter 5). Medical technologies also offered my interlocutors the option of dealing with the metabolic health complications of PCOS in the future, when these issues began to be manifested, rather than in the present through prophylactic lifestyle modifications.

Simultaneously, negotiations with intimate partners helped urban professional middle-class women offset the social consequences of PCOS-related subfertility (Chapter 6). Women with the condition would acquaint their partners with the possibility of reproductive issues and even childlessness, and they would expect their partners to be supportive as they navigated these PCOS-related issues. Although my interlocutors with PCOS often experienced deep distress as the possibility of childlessness became more tangible, they nevertheless prioritized conjugal intimacy over reproduction. Their negotiation of these expectations with their (potential) spouses allowed them to not have to worry about subfertility until they started trying to conceive.

Women also tried to navigate the possible consequences of their toxic location on general wellness, in terms of both prophylaxis and mitigation, through consumption. They engaged in precautionary consumption, aimed at preventing and reducing their exposure to pollutants, EDCs, and adulterants. They also turned toward consuming health supplements, toiletries, and personal care products that promised to tackle or reduce the effects of pollution and environmental contamination (Chapter 5). At best, their harm reduction practices functioned as token gestures that provided a sense of agency and control. Nonetheless, my interlocutors had the economic means to engage in such harm reduction, even though it could not really protect them from exposure to EDCs and other contaminants.

Toxicity and Uncertainty

The concern with pollution and contamination that motivated harm reduction practices did not, however, get channeled into collective action. Even as my interlocutors—be they women with PCOS or medical interlocutors—recognized the structural factors hampering optimum wellness, when it came to interventions to address the negative health consequences of those political–economic structures, they could not transcend the individual. Similarly, lay interlocutors commented on the defective modernization and unhealthy political–ecological changes brought by economic liberalization and implicated them in metabolic disorders such as PCOS, but they did not seek to transform those structures. Their lay epidemiology of PCOS did not manage to become a "popular epidemiology" (Brown 1992, 2007), that is, a way of knowing and talking about PCOS that was harnessed toward political ends.

Much of the social scientific literature on toxicity has highlighted difficulties in rendering toxicity perceptible and measuring its effects (e.g., Fortun and Fortun 2005; Murphy 2006; Nash 2006; Wylie 2018). Given cumulative exposures, long temporal spans to manifestation, and difficulties in defining exposure and thresholds (see Chapter 1), the exact health effects of toxicants such as EDCs are enveloped in uncertainty. Scientists, regulators, affected people, and corporations battle over this uncertainty and its political implications; various stakeholders are invested in manufacturing uncertainty whereas various others are invested in unraveling it. When it came to PCOS, my interlocutors (whether lay, medical, or with PCOS) recognized a role for rising levels of environmental contamination, EDCs, and pollutants. They blamed them for mounting PCOS incidence. This was a visceral recognition that they could not root in scientific evidence or objectivity. However, just as interlocutors were not engaged in collective action aimed at transforming the structures that they linked to PCOS vulnerability, they were not invested in rendering pollution, environmental contamination, and their effects knowable either. Such evidence gathering ventures did not command their attention. Instead, their energy was deflected into navigating their toxic location through individual harm reduction measures. Moreover, they saw their intoxication as an inescapable part of the modernity they enjoyed. When placed in that perspective, it was an acceptable consequence. Rendering its extent and effects perceptible and measurable would not change this situation.

PCOS and Toxic Worlding

What insights do these toxic worldings of urban professional middle-class women with PCOS in India have to offer? For one, they highlight again the issue of viable and desirable options when it comes to living with toxicity. When studying toxicity, we must consider the alternatives—what would a world without such toxicity look like, and what would the lives of our interlocutors look like in that world? My interlocutors were not engaging in intentional or willful intoxication as were the interlocutors of Hardon (2021) or Pine (2016), mentioned above. Nor did they see the "slow violence" (Nixon 2011) of their intoxication as a preferable alternative to lives filled with other forms of more tangible violence as was the case in Roberts's study. Rather, the toxic worldings of my interlocutors speak to an acceptable intoxication and to the pleasures upon which toxicity can be attendant; without attention to these pleasures and to the acceptance of the risks and harms involved in accessing those pleasures, we are left with an incomplete picture of living with toxicity. Toxicity can be entangled in life worlds, not just due to economic necessity, but, as the case of urban professional middle-class Indian women with PCOS shows, also as a result of the structuring of subjectivities.

Issues related to pollution and contamination are becoming ever-more salient in our current geological era, the Anthropocene, which is marked by significant human impact on the Earth's ecosystems. Scholars, activists, and lay persons alike must grapple with questions of how to deal with toxicity, reduce its harms, and effect change for the better. A particular challenge to such efforts has been the seeming resignation, apathy, or indifference toward changing toxic structures and regimes that can be expressed by the very people most affected by such structures. Sometimes, this resignation or indifference can be caused by a community's livelihoods and economic survival being embroiled with the production of toxicity (Eriksen 2018; Lora–Wainwright 2013). However, the indifference can also be the product of a sufferer's or a community's sense of a lack of agency in being able to seek redress (Lora–Wainwright 2010). If an awareness of pollution's health effects cannot be harnessed toward action from the state, then that knowledge can seem largely futile or even anxiety-provoking and hence counterproductive. Although it is difficult to say with certainty what prevented my interlocutors from seeking structural changes to address the toxicity that they experienced, it is likely that it was not only an affective investment in the advantages that it brought but also a sense of the inevitability of their toxic location.

The perpetuation of toxicity then is indelibly dependent upon the advantages, pleasures, and security that it can bring. As mentioned in Chapter 1, toxicity is not only produced by certain political–economic regimes, but it can also be reproductive of these regimes. My interlocutors with PCOS were harmed by their toxic location. They were nevertheless aiding the perpetuation of that location by functioning as the producers (as professionals and employees) and consumers (of the products and services manufactured and disposed of under poorly implemented regulations) that kept in place the larger political–economic structures that produced that location. They had been co-opted into the regimes that were also harming their health.

Toxicity, pollution, and environmental degradation have often been framed as being inevitable in the course of development, and addressing them is portrayed as antithetical to poverty alleviation and economic stability. As a result, much of the Global South faces a complicated balancing act between pursuing developmental goals (a "brown agenda") and environmental goals (a "green agenda"). Activism related to the harms of environmental toxicity, when that toxicity is not challenging immediate livelihoods, is associated with a "full belly" politics—people and communities for whom precarity and struggles for food, sleep, and shelter are daily realities cannot spare the time, attention, and other resources to think in terms of the distant future. The intriguing thing about my interlocutors, though, was that they were comfortably off. Amita Baviskar (2003) has written about a form of environmentalism emergent in India among the privileged urban classes that she terms "bourgeois environmentalism." Bourgeois environmentalism, rather than focusing on issues of social and environmental justice and resource stewardship, is preoccupied with creating bourgeois spaces that are free of polluting industries and labor. To do so, it attempts to shunt these activities and people to the margins. My research would suggest that professional middle-class harm reduction practices are also shot through with a similar logic. Rather than targeting toxic structures, such consumption-based harm reduction attempts to fortify bodily boundaries against toxicity; it aims to "cleanse" only the space enclosed within those boundaries (see also Pathak 2020). What would efforts to address toxic locations and structures look like if they managed to transcend limited, individualized attempts? Research addressing this question would have much to offer.

This book is centered on Indian women of the urban professional middle-class segment who have been diagnosed with PCOS. As mentioned in Chapter 3, this focus should not be taken to suggest that women of this class segment are the most affected by toxicity, or that women of lower socioeconomic strata in India do not experience PCOS, or that women of lower socioeconomic strata do not experience it as a disruption. The urban middle class in India is, however, the class that "sets the terms of reference of Indian society" (Jaffrelot and Van der Veer 2008: 19) when it comes to aspiration and consumption. It is also the class most affected by high rates of metabolic disorders. Initial studies and anecdotal evidence from medical practitioners suggested that PCOS prevalence was highest among this class. As mentioned in Chapter 1 and Chapter 3, however, this is likely to change with time. How is PCOS experienced and negotiated among other socioeconomic strata, especially among strata that lack easy access to medical technologies or among those whose class identity is contingent upon different gender or conjugal norms? What unique burdens contribute to PCOS vulnerability in these strata, and what are the typical constraints to management faced by those affected? Moreover, what does PCOS look like outside of India, and what can the comparative perspective teach us about better managing the condition and mitigating its harms? To truly address PCOS and to design interventions aimed at reducing its prevalence and incidence, we need more research into the various pressures faced across the life course by women not just in urban India but also in other globalizing regions with a high incidence of lifestyle diseases. Finally, PCOS is the female manifestation of a toxic location associated with modernity, aspiration, and globalization; it would be illuminating to examine the male side of this dynamic, in terms of male experiences of endocrine and metabolic issues.

Most research on toxicity has focused on members of economically and otherwise disadvantaged groups. In this book, I have used PCOS as a window into a toxic location that is not linked to a marginalized socioeconomic status in order to examine larger interactions between the health pressures of capitalist modernity and consumer globalization, environmental exploitation, and the rise of lifestyle disorders. Women of the urban professional middle-class segment in India experience unique stressors that affect their health. Those stressors are nonetheless associated with political–economic changes that bring desired identities within reach. Women's aspirations and identities are therefore simultaneously aided and constrained by the political–economic shifts that make them vulnerable to PCOS. PCOS, then, is the reflection of the ills of a regime of toxic production and consumption in the domain of reproduction. This book has examined life amid a relatively privileged, yet nevertheless toxic, location. As we are faced with the growing recognition of the human–environmental health sequelae of the Anthropocene, toxicity has the potential to congeal into a "binding crisis" (Jeffrey 2015: 815)—a crisis that transcends class boundaries and other inequalities, disrupting life enough to allow for action that is beneficial to all, whether humans or more-than-humans. For this potential to be achieved, however, energy devoted to addressing toxicity cannot be deflected through action centered on the individual.

Note

1 Testosterone is one of the most well-known androgens. As mentioned in the introduction, in popular parlance, androgens are often simplistically termed "male hormones." Such nomenclature cannot capture the more complicated reality that androgens are present across sexes, although at different levels and in different proportions in relation to other hormones.

BIBLIOGRAPHY

Abeyasekera, Asha. 2016. Narratives of Choice: Marriage, Choosing Right and the Responsibility of Agency in Urban Middle-Class Sri Lanka. *Feminist Review* 113(1): 1–16.

Acharya, A., V. P. Reddaiah, and N. Baridalyne. 2006. Nutritional Status and Menarche in Adolescent Girls in an Urban Resettlement Colony of South Delhi. *Indian Journal of Community Medicine* 31(4): 302–303.

Agard–Jones, Vanessa. 2013. Bodies in the System. *Small Axe* 17(3): 182–192.

Agrawal, Anju, Ravi S. Pandey, and Bechan Sharma. 2010. Water Pollution with Special Reference to Pesticide Contamination in India. *Journal of Water Resource and Protection* 2(5): 432–448.

Agrawal, Binod C. 1997. The Meanings of Hinglishness: Liberalisation and Globalisation in Indian Broadcasting. In *Programming for People: From Cultural Rights to Cultural Responsibilities*. Kevin Robins, ed. Pp. 144–155, Vol. Nov 19–21. New York: United Nations World Television Forum.

Agrawal, Praween. 2005. Role of Lifestyle and Diet in Emerging Obesity among Indian Women and Its Impact upon Their Health Status. Paper presented at the *IUSSP XXV International Population Conference Tours*, France, Jul 18.

Ahearn, Laura. 2001. *Invitations to Love: Literacy, Love letters, and Social Change in Nepal*. Ann Arbor: University of Michigan Press.

Ah-King, Malin and Eva Hayward. 2014. Toxic Sexes—Perverting Pollution and Queering Hormone Disruption. *O-Zone: A Journal of Object-Oriented Studies* 1: 1–12.

Alcoff, Linda Martín. 2006. *Visible Identities, Race, Gender, and the Self*. New York: Oxford University Press.

Aljazeera. 2009. Private Tuition Soars in India. *Aljazeera* (online), Jul 11. https://www.aljazeera.com/news/2009/7/11/private-tuition-soars-in-india, accessed Feb 7, 2021.

Amsterdam ESHRE/ASRM-Sponsored 3rd PCOS Consensus Workshop Group. 2012. Consensus on Women's Health Aspects of Polycystic Ovary Syndrome (PCOS). *Human Reproduction* 27(1): 14–24.

Anjana, R. M., R. Pradeepa, M. Deepa, M. Datta, R. Unnikrishnan, M. Rema, and V. Mohan. 2011. The Need for Obtaining Accurate Nationwide Estimates of Diabetes Prevalence in India–Rationale for a National Study on Diabetes. *Indian Journal of Medical Research* 133(4): 369–380.

Arnold, David. 2000. *Science, Technology and Medicine in Colonial India. The New Cambridge History of India*. Cambridge: Cambridge University Press.

Aronowitz, Robert. 2009. The Converged Experience of Risk and Disease. *The Milbank Quarterly* 87(2): 417–442.

Ashbacher, Kirstin, Aoife O'Donovan, Owen M. Wolkowitz, Firdaus S. Dhabhar, Yali Su, and Elissa Epel. 2013. Good Stress, Bad Stress and Oxidative Stress: Insights from Anticipatory Cortisol Reactivity. *Psychoneuroendocrinology* 38(9): 1698–1708.

Baer, Hans. 1996. Towards a Political Ecology of Health in Medical Anthropology. *Medical Anthropology Quarterly* 10(4): 451–454.

Bagga, Amrita and Shaunak Kulkarni. 2000. Age at Menarche and Secular Trend in Maharashtrian (Indian) Girls. *Acta Biologica Szegediensis* 44(1–4): 53–57.

Balen, Adam and Anthony J. Rutherford. 2007. Managing Anovulatory Infertility and Polycystic Ovary Syndrome. *British Medical Journal* 335: 663.

Balen, Adam, Roy Homburg, and Stephen Franks. 2009. Defining Polycystic Ovary Syndrome. *The British Medical Journal* 338: a2968.

van Balen, Frank and Marcia Inhorn. 2002. Interpreting Infertility: A View from the Social Sciences. In *Infertility Around the Globe: New Thinking on Childlessness, Gender, and Reproductive Technologies*. Marcia Inhorn and Frank van Balen, eds. Pp. 3–32. Berkeley: University of California Press.

Barber, T. M. and S. Franks. 2019. Chapter 27—Genetic and Environmental Factors in the Etiology of Polycystic Ovary Syndrome. In *The Ovary*. Peter C. K. Leung and Eli Y. Adashi, eds. Pp. 437–459. Academic Press. https://www.sciencedirect.com/science/article/pii/B9780128132098000273

Baru, Rama Vaidyanathan. 2000. Privatisation and Corporatisation. *Seminar* 489: 29–33.

Baviskar, Amita. 2003. Between Violence and Desire: Space, Power, and Identity in the Making of Metropolitan Delhi. *International Social Science Journal* 55: 89–98.

Beck, Ulrich. 1989. On the Way to the Industrial Risk-Society? Outline of an Argument. *Thesis Eleven* 23: 86–103.

Beck, Ulrich. 1992. *Risk Society: Towards a New Modernity*. London: Sage Publications.

Beck, Ulrich. 1999. *World Risk Society*. Cambridge: Polity Press.

Beck, Ulrich, Anthony Giddens, and Scott Lash. 1994. *Reflexive Modernization. Politics, Tradition, and Aesthetics in the Modern Social Order*. Stanford: Stanford University Press.

Beck, Ulrich and Elisabeth Beck-Gernsheim. 1995. *The Normal Chaos of Love*. Cambridge: Polity Press.

Bedi, J. S., J. P. S. Gill, R. S. Aulakh, P. Kaur, A. Sharma, and P. A. Pooni. 2013. Pesticide Residues in Human Breast Milk: Risk Assessment for Infants from Punjab, India. *Science of the Total Environment* 463–464: 720–726.

Bell, Susan E. and Anne E. Figert. 2010. Gender and the Medicalization of Healthcare. In *Palgrave Handbook of Gender and Healthcare*. Ellen Kuhlmann and Ellen Annandale, eds. Pp. 127–142. London: Palgrave Macmillan.

Benson, S., P. Arck, S. Tan, S. Hahn, K. Mann, N. Rifaie, O. Janssen, M. Schedlowski, and S. Elsenbruch. 2009. Disturbed Stress Responses in Women with Polycystic Ovary Syndrome. *Psychoneuroendocrinology* 34(5): 727–735.

Bergman, Åke, Jerrold J. Heindel, Susan Jobling, Karen A. Kidd, and R. Thomas Zoeller. 2013. *State of the Science of Endocrine Disrupting Chemicals 2012: Summary for Decision-Makers*. Geneva: World Health Organization.

Béteille, André. 1992. Caste and Family: In Representations of Indian Society. *Anthropology Today* 8(1): 13–18.

Bharadwaj, Aditya. 2000. How Some Indian Baby Makers Are Made: Media Narratives and Assisted Conception in India. *Anthropology and Medicine* 7(1): 63–78.

Bharadwaj, Aditya. 2003. Why Adoption Is Not an Option in India: The Visibility of Infertility, the Secrecy of Donor Insemination, and Other Cultural Complexities. *Social Science & Medicine* 56(9): 1867–1880.

Bharadwaj, Aditya. 2016. *Conceptions: Infertility and Procreative Technologies in India*. New York: Berghahn Books.

Bharathi, Divya and G. P. Dinesh. 2018. Women's Perspective Towards Health and Fitness—A Case Study on Indian Fitness Industry and Women. *Sumedha Journal of Management* 7(2): 229–240.

Bhasin, Sanjiv, Rahul Sharma, and N. K. Saini. 2010. Depression, Anxiety and Stress Among Adolescent Students Belonging to Affluent Families: A School-based Study. *Indian Journal of Pediatrics* 77(2): 161–165.

Bhatnagar, V. K., J. S. Patel, M. R. Variya, K. Venkaiah, M. P. Shah, and S. K. Kashyap. 1992. Levels of Organochlorine Insecticides in Human Blood from Ahmedabad (Rural), India. *Bulletin of Environmental Contamination and Toxicology* 48(2): 302–307.

Björntorp, Per, Göran Holm, Bo Jacobsson, Kristina Schiller-de Jounge, Per-Arne Lundberg, Lars Sjöström, Ulf Smith, and Lars Sullivan. 1977. Physical Training in Human Hyperplastic Obesity. IV. Effects on the Hormonal Status. *Metabolism* 26(3): 319–328.

Bode, Maarten. 2008. *Taking Traditional Knowledge to the Market: The Modern Image of the Ayurvedic and Unani Industry 1980–2000*. Hyderabad: Orient Blackswan.

Bordo, Susan. 1993. *Unbearable Weight: Feminism, Western Culture, and the Body*. Berkeley and Los Angeles: University of California Press.

Brown, Phil. 1992. Popular Epidemiology and Toxic Waste Contamination: Lay and Professional Ways of Knowing. *Journal of Health and Social Behavior* 33(3): 267–281.

Brown, Phil. 2007. *Toxic Exposures. Contested Illnesses and the Environmental Health Movement*. New York: Columbia University Press.

Bushnik, Tracey, Douglas Haines, Patrick Levallois, Johanne Levesque, Jay van Oostdam, and Claude Viau. 2010. Lead and Bisphenol A Concentrations in the Canadian Population. *Health Reports* 21(3): 7–18.

Butler, Judith. 1990. *Gender Trouble: Feminism and the Subversion of Identity*. New York: Routledge.

Butler, Judith. 1993. *Bodies That Matter. On the Discursive Limits of Sex*. New York: Routledge.

Carpenter, David O. 2006. Polychlorinated Biphenyls (PCBs): Routes of Exposure and Effects on Human Health. *Reviews on Environmental Health* 21(1): 1–23.

Carré, Julie, Nicolas Gatimel, Jessika Moreau, Jean Parinaud, and Roger Léandri. 2017. Does Air Pollution Play a Role in Infertility?: A Systematic Review. *Environmental Health* 16: 82.

Celermajer, David, Clara Chow, Eloi Marijon, Nicholas Anstey, and Kam Woo. 2012. Cardiovascular Disease in the Developing World: Prevalences, Patterns, and the Potential of Early Disease Detection. *Journal of the American College of Cardiology* 60(14): 1207–1216.

Chakrabarty, Dipesh. 2008. *Provincializing Europe: Postcolonial Thought and Historical Difference*. Princeton and Oxford: Princeton University Press.

Chakraborty, Paromita, Sanjenbam Nirmala Khuman, Bhupandar Kumar, and Bommanna Loganathan. 2017. HCH and DDT Residues in Indian Soil: Atmospheric Input and Risk Assessment. In *Xenobiotics in the Soil Environment: Monitoring, Toxicity, and Management*. M. Hashmi, V. Kumar, and A. Varma, eds. Pp. 21–40. Cham: Springer.

Chatterjee, Partha. 1986. *Nationalist Thought and the Colonial World: A Derivative Discourse*. New Delhi: Oxford University Press.

Chatterjee, Partha. 1993. *The Nation and Its Fragments: Colonial and Postcolonial Histories*. Princeton: Princeton University Press.

Checker, Melissa. 2007. "But I Know It's True": Environmental Risk Assessment, Justice, and Anthropology. *Human Organization* 66(2): 112–124.

Chopra, S. M., A. Misra, S. Gulati, and R. Gupta. 2013. Overweight, Obesity and Related Non-Communicable Diseases in Asian Indian Girls and Women. *European Journal of Clinical Nutrition* 67: 688–696.

Cielemęcka, Olga and Cecilia Åsberg. 2019. Introduction. *Environmental Humanities* 11(1): 101–107.

Conforti, Alessandro, Marika Mascia, Giuseppina Cioffi, Cristina De Angelis, Giuseppe Coppola, Pasquale De Rosa, Rosario Pivonello, Carlo Alviggi, and Giuseppe De Placido. 2018. Air Pollution and Female Fertility: A systematic Review of Literature. *Reproductive Biology and Endocrinology* 16: 117.

Connolly, V., N. Unwin, P. Sherriff, R. Bilous, and W. Kelly. 2000. Diabetes Prevalence and Socioeconomic Status: A Population Based Study Showing Increased Prevalence of Type 2 Diabetes Mellitus in Deprived Areas. *Journal of Epidemiology & Community Health* 54: 173–177.

Conrad, Peter. 1992. Medicalization and Social Control. *Annual Review of Sociology* 18: 209–232.

Corea, Gena. 1985. *The Mother Machine: Reproductive Technologies from Artificial Insemination to Artificial Wombs*. New York: Harper and Row Publishers.

Cullity, Jocelyn. 2002. The Global Desi: Cultural Nationalism on MTV India. *Journal of Communication Inquiry* 26(4): 408–425.

Cussons, Andrea, Bronwyn Stuckey, John P. Walsh, Valerie Burke, and Robert Norman. 2005. Polycystic Ovarian Syndrome: Marked Differences Between Endocrinologists and Gynaecologists in Diagnosis and Management. *Clinical Endocrinology* 62(3): 289–295.

Dambhare, Dharampal, Sanjay Wagh, and Jayesh Dudhe. 2012. Age at Menarche and Menstrual Cycle Pattern among School Adolescent Girls in Central India. *Global Journal of Health Science* 4(1): 105–111.

Darbre, Philippa D. 2018. Overview of Air Pollution and Endocrine Disorders. *International Journal of General Medicine* 11: 191–207.

Davis, Coralynn V. 2009. Im/possible Lives: Gender, Class, Self-Fashioning, and Affinal Solidarity in Modern South Asia. *Social Identities* 15(2): 243–272.

Davison, Charlie, George Davey Smith, and Stephen Frankel. 1991. Lay Epidemiology and the Prevention Paradox: The Implications of Coronary Candidacy for Health Education. *Sociology of Health & Illness* 13(1): 1–19.

Deb, Sibnath, Pooja Chatterjee, and Kerryann Walsh. 2010. Anxiety among High School Students in India: Comparisons Across Gender, School Type, Social Strata and Perceptions of Quality Time with Parents. *Australian Journal of Educational and Developmental Psychology* 10(1): 18–31.

Delemarre-Van de Waal, H. A. 2005. Secular Trend of Timing of Puberty. In *Abnormalities in Puberty: Scientific and Clinical Advances*. H. A. Delemarre-Van de Waal, ed. Pp. 1–14. Basel: Karger.

Desai, P., V. Shrinivasan, and M. Hazra.1992. Understanding the Emotions of Infertile Couples. *Journal of Obstetrics and Gynaecology of India* 42: 498–503.

Deshpande, Satish. 2003. *Contemporary India: A Sociological View*. New York: Viking.

Desjarlais, Robert and C. Jason Throop. 2011. Phenomenological Approaches in Anthropology. *Annual Review of Anthropology* 40: 87–102.

Dhaliwal, L. K., K. R. Khera, and G. I. Dhall. 1991. Evaluation and Two-Year Follow-Up of 455 Infertile Couples—Pregnancy Rate and Outcome. *International Journal of Fertility* 36(4): 222–226.

Dhillon, Megha and Priti Dhawan. 2011. "But I Am Fat": The Experiences of Weight Dissatisfaction in Indian Adolescent Girls and Young Women. *Women's Studies International Forum* 34(6): 539–549.

Di Chiro, Giovanna. 2010. Polluted Politics? Confronting Toxic Discourse, Sex Panic, and Eco-Normativity. In *Queer Ecologies: Sex, Nature, Politics, Desire*. Catriona Mortimer-Sandilands and Bruce Erickson, eds. Pp. 199–230. Bloomington: Indiana University Press.

Diamanti-Kandarakis, Evanthia, Jean-Pierre Bourguignon, Linda C. Giudice, Russ Hauser, Gail S. Prins, Ana M. Soto, R. Thomas Zoeller, and Andrea C. Gore. 2009. Endocrine-Disrupting Chemicals: An Endocrine Society Scientific Statement. *Endocrine Reviews* 30(4): 293–342.

Diamond, Jared. 2011. Diabetes in India. *Nature* 469: 478–479.

Dickey, Sara. 2002. Anjali's Prospects: Class Mobility in Urban India. In *Everyday Life in South Asia*. Diane P. Mines and Sarah Lamb, eds. Pp. 214–226. Bloomington: Indiana University Press.

Donner, Henrike. 2002. "One's Own Marriage": Love Marriages in a Calcutta Neighbourhood. *South Asia Research* 22(1): 79–94.

Donner, Henrike. 2003. The Place of Birth: Childbearing and Kinship in Calcutta Middle-Class Families. *Medical Anthropology* 22(4): 303–341.

Donner, Henrike. 2006. Committed Mothers and Well-Adjusted Children: Privatisation, Early-Years Education and Motherhood in Calcutta. *Modern Asian Studies* 40(2): 371–395.

Donner, Henrike. 2008. *Domestic Goddesses: Maternity, Globalization, and Middle-Class Identity in Contemporary India*. London and New York: Routledge.

Donner, Henrike. 2011. *Being Middle-Class in India: A Way of Life*. New York: Routledge.

Donner, Henrike. 2016. Doing It Our Way: Love and Marriage in Kolkata Middle-Class Families. *Modern Asian Studies* 50(4): 1147–1189.

Donner, Henrike and Geert de Neve. 2011. Introduction. In *Being Middle-Class in India: A Way of Life*. Henrike Donner, ed. Pp. 1–22. New York: Routledge.

Donner, Henrike and Gonçalo Santos. 2016. Love, Marriage, and Intimate Citizenship in Contemporary China and India: An Introduction. *Modern Asian Studies* 50(4): 1123–1146.

Dwyer, Rachel. 2011. Zara Hatke ('Somewhat Different'): The New Middle Classes and the Changing Forms of Hindi Cinema. In *Being Middle-Class in India: A Way of Life*. Henrike Donner, ed. Pp. 184–208. New York: Routledge.

Eagleton, Terry. 1990. *The Significance of Theory*. Cambridge: Blackwell.

Eckel, Robert H., Scott M. Grundy, and Paul Z. Zimmet. 2005. The Metabolic Syndrome. *The Lancet* 365(9468): 1415–1428.

Ecks, Stefan. 2010. Spectacles of Reason: An Ethnography of Indian Gastroenterologists. In *Technologized Images, Technologized Bodies*. Jeannette Edwards, Penny Harvey, and Peter Wade, eds. Pp. 117–135. Oxford: Bergahn Books.

Economic Times. 2011. How the Indian Economy Changed in 1991-2011. *Economic Times*, Jul 24. https://economictimes.indiatimes.com/news/economy/indicators/how-the-indian-economy-changed-in-1991-2011/articleshow/9339258.cms, accessed Jun 26, 2021.

Economist. 2008. India and Pollution: Up to Their Necks in It. *Economist* 388(8589). http://www.economist.com/node/11751397, accessed Jul 8, 2014.

Ehrmann, David. 2005. Polycystic Ovary Syndrome. *New England Journal of Medicine* 352(12): 1223–1236.

Ehrmann, David A., David R. Liljenquist, Kristen Kasza, Ricardo Azziz, Richard S. Legro, and Mahmoud N. Ghazzi. 2006. Prevalence and Predictors of the Metabolic Syndrome in Women with Polycystic Ovary Syndrome. *The Journal of Clinical Endocrinology & Metabolism* 91(1): 48–53.

Enas, Enas A., Vishwanathan Mohan, Mohan Deepa, Syed Farooq, Suraj Pazhoor, and Hancy Chennikkara. 2007. The Metabolic Syndrome and Dyslipidemia among Asian Indians: A Population with High Rates of Diabetes and Premature Coronary Artery Disease. *The Journal of the Cardiometabolic Syndrome* 2(4): 267–275.

Eriksen, Thomas Hylland. 2018. Scales of Environmental Engagement in an Industrial Town: Glocal Perspectives from Gladstone, Queensland. *Ethnos* 83(3): 423–439.

Everson, Susan, Debbie E. Goldberg, Susan P. Helmrich, Timo A. Lakka, John W. Lynch, George A. Kaplan, and Jukka T. Salonen. 1998. Weight Gain and the Risk of Developing Insulin Resistance. *Diabetes Care* 21(10): 1637–1643.

Farmer, Paul. 1988. Bad Blood, Spoiled Milk: Bodily Fluids as Moral Barometers in Rural Haiti. *American Ethnologist* 15(1): 62–83.

Farmer, Paul. 1999. *Infections and Inequalities: The Modern Plague*. Berkeley: University of California Press.

Fee, Margery. 2006. Racializing Narratives: Obesity, Diabetes and the "Aboriginal" Thrifty Genotype. *Social Science & Medicine* 62(12): 2988–2997.

Fee, Elizabeth and Nancy Krieger. 1993. Understanding AIDS: Historical Interpretations and the Limits of Biomedical Individualism. *American Journal of Public Health* 83(10): 1477–1486.

Fernandes, Leela. 2000a. Nationalizing "the Global": Media Images, Cultural Politics and the Middle Class in India. *Media, Culture & Society* 22(5): 611–628.

Fernandes, Leela. 2000b. Restructuring the New Middle Class in Liberalizing India. *Comparative Studies of South Asia, Africa, and the Middle East* 20(1&2): 88–104.

Fernandes, Leela. 2001. Rethinking Globalization. Gender and the Nation in India. In *Feminist Locations. Global and Local, Theory and Practice*. Marianne Dekoven, ed. Pp. 147–167. New Brunswick: Rutgers University Press.

Fernandes, Leela. 2006. *India's New Middle Class: Democratic Politics in an Era of Reform*. Minneapolis: University of Minnesota Press.

Fernandes, Leela and Patrick Heller. 2006. Hegemonic Aspirations: New Middle Class Politics and India's Democracy in Comparative Perspective. *Critical Asian Studies* 38(4): 495–522.

Fortun, Kim and Mike Fortun. 2005. Scientific Imaginaries and Ethical Plateaus in Contemporary U.S. Toxicology. *American Anthropologist* 107(1): 43–54.

Franks, Stephen. 1995. Polycystic Ovary Syndrome. *New England Journal of Medicine* 333: 853–861.

Frickel, Scott. 2004. *Chemical Consequences: Environmental Mutagens, Scientist Activism, and the Rise of Genetic Toxicology.* New Brunswick: Rutgers University Press.

Friedman, Sara. 2006. *Intimate Politics: Marriage, the Market and State Power in Southeastern China.* Cambridge: Harvard University Press.

Fuller, Christopher J. and Haripriya Narasimhan. 2008. Companionate Marriage in India: The Changing Marriage System in a Middle-Class Brahman Subcaste. *Journal of the Royal Anthropological Institute* 14(4): 736–754.

Gaiha, Raghav, Raghbendra Jha, and Vani S. Kulkarni. 2013. How Pervasive Is Eating Out in India? *Journal of Asian and African Studies* 48(3): 370–386.

Gamper-Rabindran, Shanti and Shreyasi Jha. 2004. Environmental Impact of India's Trade Liberalization. *Social Science Research Network.* https://ssrn.com/abstract=574161, accessed Jan 21, 2021.

Ganguly–Scrase, Ruchira. 2003. Paradoxes of Globalization, Liberalization, and Gender Equality: The Worldviews of the Lower Middle Class in West Bengal, India. *Gender & Society* 17(4): 544–566.

Garari, Kaniza. 2014. PCOS—All You Need to Know. *Asian Age* (online), Jun 30. http://www.pressreader.com/india/the-asian-age/20140630/283304635608094, accessed Feb 24, 2021.

Geissler, P. Wenzel and Ruth J. Prince. 2020. "Toxic Worldings." Introduction to Toxic Flows. *Anthropology Today* 36(6): 3–4.

Ghosh, Jayati. 2009. Tuition Culture. *Frontline* (online), 26(22), Oct 24–Nov 6. https://frontline.thehindu.com/columns/article30185206.ece, accessed Feb 6, 2021.

Giddens, Anthony. 1990. *The Consequences of Modernity.* Stanford: Stanford University Press.

Giddens, Anthony. 1991. *Modernity and Self-Identity: Self and Society in the Late Modern Age.* Stanford: Stanford University Press.

Giddens, Anthony. 1992. *The Transformation of Intimacy: Sexuality, Love and Eroticism in Modern Societies.* Stanford: Stanford University Press.

Giddens, Anthony. 1999. Risk and Responsibility. *Modern Law Review* 62(1): 1–10.

Giddens, Anthony and Christopher Pierson. 1998. *Conversations with Anthony Giddens: Making Sense of Modernity.* Oxford: Polity Press.

Gilbertson, Amanda. 2014a. A Fine Balance: Negotiating Fashion and Respectable Femininity in Middle-Class Hyderabad, India. *Modern Asian Studies* 48(1): 120–158.

Gilbertson, Amanda. 2014b. From Respect to Friendship? Companionate Marriage and Conjugal Power Negotiation in Middle-Class Hyderabad. *South Asia: Journal of South Asian Studies* 37(2): 225–238.

Gillespie, Marie and Tom Cheesman. 2002. Media Cultures in India and the South Asian Diaspora. *Contemporary South Asia* 11(2): 127–133.

Globalization and World Cities Research Network. 2012. The World According to GaWC 2012. *Globalization and World Cities Research Network.* https://www.lboro.ac.uk/gawc/world2012t.html, accessed Jul 6, 2021.

Gold, Ann Grodzins. 1998. Sin and Rain: Moral Ecology in Rural North India. In *Purifying the Earthly Body of God: Religion and Ecology in Hindu India.* Lance E. Nelson, ed. Pp. 165–195. Albany: State University of New York Press.

Good, Byron J. 1977. The Heart of What's the Matter: The Semantics of Illness in Iran. *Culture, Medicine, and Psychiatry* 1: 25–58.

Goodman, Alan H. 2000. When Genes Don't Count (for Racial Differences in Health). *American Journal of Public Health* 90(11): 1699–1702.

Goran, Michael I. and Barbara A. Gower. 2001. Longitudinal Study on Pubertal Insulin Resistance. *Diabetes* 50(11): 2444–2450.

Gouri, Venugopal. 2012. Confront the Condition. *Hindu*, Dec 4.

Greenstone, Michael and Rohini Pande. 2014. India's Particulate Problem. *The New York Times*, Feb 9.

Griffiths, Paula L. and Margaret Bentley. 2001. The Nutrition Transition Is Underway in India. *The Journal of Nutrition* 131(10): 2692–2700.

Gujral, Unjali, R. Pradeepa, Mary Beth Weber, K. M. Venkat Narayan, and Vishwanathan Mohan. 2013. Type 2 Diabetes in South Asians: Similarities and Differences with White Caucasian and Other Populations. *Annals of the New York Academy of Sciences* 1281(1): 51–63.

Gulati, Seema and Anoop Misra. 2014. Sugar Intake, Obesity, and Diabetes in India. *Nutrients* 6(12): 5955–5974.

Gupta, Jyotsna Agnihotri. 2000. *New Reproductive Technologies, Women's Health and Autonomy: Freedom or Dependency?* New Delhi: Sage Publications.

Gupta, Priyanka K. 2004. Pesticide Exposure—Indian Scene. *Toxicology* 198(1–3): 83–90.

Gupta, R., V. P. Gupta, M. Sarna, H. Prakash, S. Rastogi, and K. D. Gupta. 2003. Serial Epidemiological Surveys in an Urban Indian Population Demonstrate Increasing Coronary Risk Factors among the Lower Socioeconomic Strata. *The Journal of the Association of Physicians of India* 51: 470–477.

Guthman, Julie. 2012. Opening Up the Black Box of the Body in Geographical Obesity Research: Toward a Critical Political Ecology of Fat. *Annals of the Association of American Geographers* 102(5): 951–957.

Guthman, Julie. 2013. Too Much Food and Too Little Sidewalk? Problematizing the Obesogenic Environment Thesis. *Environment and Planning A* 45(1): 142–158.

H. T. Correspondents. 2013. How Air and Water Pollution Plagues Indian Cities. *Hindustan Times*, Dec 1.

Hacking, Ian. 1999. *The Social Construction of What?* Cambridge: Harvard University Press.

Halliburton, Murphy. 2004. Finding a Fit: Psychiatric Pluralism in South India and Its Implications for WHO Studies of Mental Disorder. *Transcultural Psychiatry* 41(1): 80–98.

Halliburton, Murphy. 2005. "Just Some Spirits": The Erosion of Spirit Possession and the Rise of "Tension" in South India. *Medical Anthropology* 24(2): 111–144.

Hankey, Alex. 2005. The Scientific Value of Ayurveda. *The Journal of Alternative and Complementary Medicine* 11(2): 221–225.

Hansen, Thomas Blom. 2001. *Violence in Urban India: Identity Politics, "Mumbai," and the Postcolonial City*. Delhi: Permanent Black.

Haraway, Donna. 1991 [1985]. A Cyborg Manifesto: Science, Technology, and Socialist-Feminism in the Late Twentieth Century. In *Simians, Cyborgs, and Women: The Reinvention of Nature*. Pp. 149–181. New York: Routledge.

Hardon, Anita. 2021. *Chemical Youth. Navigating Uncertainty in Search of the Good Life*. Cham: Palgrave Macmillan.

Harris, Gardiner. 2014. Cities in India among the Most Polluted, W.H.O. Says. *The New York Times*, May 8.

Hashmi, Tanveer Alam, Rizwana Qureshi, Devayani Tipre, and Shobhana Menon. 2020. Investigation of Pesticide Residues in Water, Sediments and Fish Samples from Tapi River, India, as a Case Study and Its Forensic Significance. *Environmental Forensics* 21(1): 1–10.

Hawkes, Corinna. 2006. Uneven Dietary Development: Linking the Policies and Processes of Globalization with the Nutrition Transition, Obesity and Diet-Related Chronic Diseases. *Global Health* 2(4): 1–18.

Hirsch, Jennifer S. and Holly Wardlow (eds.). 2006. *Modern Loves: The Anthropology of Romantic Courtship and Companionate Marriage*. Ann Arbor: University of Michigan Press.

Holmes, Seth. 2011. Structural Vulnerability and Hierarchies of Ethnicity and Citizenship on the Farm. *Medical Anthropology* 30(4): 425–449.

Homburg, Roy. 2006. Pregnancy Complications in PCOS. *Best Practice & Research Clinical Endocrinology & Metabolism* 20(2): 281–292.

Inden, Ronald B. 1990. *Imagining India*. Oxford: Blackwell.

India State-Level Disease Burden Initiative Diabetes Collaborators. 2018. The Increasing Burden of Diabetes and Variations among the States of India: The Global Burden of Disease Study 1990–2016. *The Lancet: Global Health* 6(12): e1352–e1362.

Inhorn, Marcia C. 2015. *Cosmopolitan Conceptions: IVF Sojourns in Global Dubai*. Durham and London: Duke University Press.

Inhorn, Marcia C. and Aditya Bharadwaj. 2007. "Reproductively Disabled Lives: Infertility, Stigma, and Suffering in Egypt and India." In *Disability in Local and Global Worlds*. Benedicte Ingstad and Susan R. Whyte, eds. Pp. 78–106. Berkeley: University of California Press.

IQAir. 2020a. World's Most Polluted Cities 2019 (PM2.5). *IQAir*. https://www.iqair.com/world-most-polluted-cities?continent=&country=&state=&page=1&perPage=50&cities=, accessed Jun 5, 2020.

IQAir. 2020b. World's Most Polluted Countries 2019 (PM2.5). *IQAir*. https://www.iqair.com/world-most-polluted-countries, accessed Jun 5, 2020.

Jacobson, Doranne. 1982. Studying the Changing Roles of Women in Rural India. *Signs* 8(1): 132–137.

Jacubowicz, D., M. Barnea, J. Wainstein, and O. Froy. 2013. Effects of Caloric Intake Timing on Insulin Resistance and Hyperandrogenism in Lean Women with Polycystic Ovary Syndrome. *Clinical Science* 125(9): 423–432.

Jaffrelot, Christopher and Peter van der Veer. 2008. Introduction. In *Patterns of Middle Class Consumption in India and China*. Christopher Jaffrelot and Peter van der Veer, eds. Pp. 11–34. New Delhi: Sage Publications.

Jamieson, Lynn. 1999. Intimacy Transformed? A Critical Look at the "Pure Relationship". *Sociology* 33(3): 477–494.

Jeffery, Roger. 1988. *The Politics of Health in India*. Berkeley: University of California Press.

Jeffery, Patricia, Roger Jeffery, and Andrew Lyon. 1989. *Labour Pains and Labour Power: Women and Childbearing in India*. London: Zed Books.

Jeffrey, Robin. 2015. Clean India! Symbols, Policies, and Tensions. *South Asia: Journal of South Asian Studies* 38(4): 807–819.

Jejeebhoy, Shireen. 1998. Infertility in India: Levels, Patterns and Consequences Priorities for Social Science Research. *Journal of Family Welfare* 44: 15–24.

Jindal, U. N. and A. N. Gupta. 1989. Social Problems of Infertile Women in India. *International Journal of Fertility* 34(1): 30–33.

John, Mary E. 1998. Globalisation, Sexuality and the Visual Field. Issues and Non-Issues for Cultural Critique. In *A Question of Silence: The Sexual Economics of Modern India.* Mary John and Janaki Nair, eds. Pp. 368–396. New Delhi: Kali for Women.

Jordan, Brigitte. 1993 [1978]. *Birth in Four Cultures: A Crosscultural Investigation of Childbirth in Yucatan, Holland, Sweden, and the United States.* Prospect Heights: Waveland.

Joshi, Beena, Srabani Mukherjee, Anushree Patil, Ameya Purandare, Sanjay Chauhan, and Rama Vaidya. 2014. A Cross-Sectional Study of Polycystic Ovarian Syndrome among Adolescent and Young Girls in Mumbai, India. *Indian Journal of Endocrinology and Metabolism* 18(3): 317–324.

Kalra, Sanjay and Ambika Gopalkrishnan Unnikrishnan. 2012. Obesity in India: The Weight of the Nation. *Journal of Medical Nutrition and Nutraceuticals* 1(1): 37–41.

Kandaraki, Eleni, Antonis Chatzigeorgiou, Sarantis Livadas, Eleni Palioura, Frangiscos Economou, Michael Koutsilieris, Sotiria Palimeri, Dimitrios Panidis, and Evanthia Diamanti-Kandarakis. 2011. Endocrine Disruptors and Polycystic Ovary Syndrome (PCOS): Elevated Serum Levels of Bisphenol A in Women with PCOS. *The Journal of Clinical Endocrinology & Metabolism* 96(3): E480–E484.

Kang, Xuezhi, Lina Jia, and Xueyong Shen. 2015. Manifestation of Hyperandrogenism in the Continuous Light Exposure-Induced PCOS Rat Model. *BioMed Research International.* https://www.hindawi.com/journals/bmri/2015/943694/

Kannuri, Nanda Kishor and Sushrut Jadhav. 2018. Generating Toxic Landscapes: Impact on Well-Being of Cotton Farmers in Telangana, India. *Anthropology & Medicine* 25(2): 121–140.

Kasbekar, Asha. 2006. *Pop Culture India!: Media, Arts, and Lifestyle.* Santa Barbara, CA: ABC-CLIO.

Kasl, Stanislav V. 1984. Stress and Health. *Annual Review of Public Health* 5: 319–341.

Kaur, Ravinder and Rajni Palriwala (eds.). 2014. *Marrying in South Asia: Shifting Concepts, Changing Practices in a Globalising World.* New Delhi: Orient Blackswan.

Khadilkar, V. V., R. Stanhope, and V. Khadilkar. 2006. Secular Trends in Puberty. *Indian Pediatrics* 43: 475–478.

Khandelwal, S. and K. S. Reddy. 2013. Eliciting a Policy Response for the Rising Epidemic of Overweight–Obesity in India. *Obesity Reviews* 14(Suppl. 2): 114–125.

Khanna, Geeta and Satwanti Kapoor. 2004. Secular Trend in Stature and Age at Menarche among Punjabi Aroras Residing in New Delhi, India. *Coolegium Anthropologicum* 28(2): 571–575.

Khosla, Ishi. 2009. Beating PCOS. *Indian Express,* May 10. https://indianexpress.com/article/news-archive/web/beating-pcos/, accessed Feb 24, 2021.

Kim, Jim Young, Joyce Millen, Alec Irwin, and John Gershman (eds.). 2000. *Dying for Growth: Global Inequality and the Health of the Poor.* Monroe: Common Courage Press.

Kitzinger, Celia and Jo Willmott. 2002. "The Thief of Womanhood": Women's Experience of Polycystic Ovarian Syndrome. *Social Science & Medicine* 54(3): 349–361.

Kleinman, Arthur. 1986. *Social Origins of Distress and Disease: Depression, Neurasthenia, and Pain in Modern China*. New Haven: Yale University Press.

Kohli, Atul. 2006. Politics of Economic Growth in India, 1980-2005. Part II: The 1990s and Beyond. *Economic and Political Weekly* 41(14): 1361–1370.

Kohli-Khandekar, Vanita. 2010. *The Indian Media Business*. New Delhi: Sage Publications.

Krieger, Nancy. 1994. Epidemiology and the Web of Causation: Has Anyone Seen the Spider? *Social Science & Medicine* 39(7): 887–903.

Krieger, Nancy. 2001. Theories for Social Epidemiology in the 21st Century: An Ecosocial Approach. *International Journal of Epidemiology* 30(4): 668–677.

Kumar, Meenakshi. 2007. Growing Pains: Now, Teenagers Affected by PCOS Problem. *Times of India*, Jun 24. https://timesofindia.indiatimes.com/india/Growing-pains-Now-teenagers-affected-by-PCOS-problem/articleshow/2144319.cms, accessed Feb 24, 2021.

Kumar, Nita. 2020. Indian Modernity as the Problem of Indian Education. In *Elementary Education in India: Policy Shifts, Issues, and Challenges*. Jyoti Raina, ed. Pp. 122–134. Abingdon: Routledge.

Kurzrock, Razelle and Philip R. Cohen. 2007. Polycystic Ovary Syndrome in Men: Stein–Leventhal Syndrome Revisited. *Medical Hypotheses* 68(3): 480–483.

Langston, Nancy. 2010. *Toxic Bodies: Hormone Disruptors and the Legacy of DES*. New Haven: Yale University Press.

Leeder, Stephen, Susan Raymond, Henry Greenberg, Hui Liu, and Kathy Esson. 2004. *A Race Against Time: The Challenge of Cardiovascular Disease in Developing Countries*. New York: Trustees of Columbia University.

Legro, R. S., A. R. Kunselman, W. C. Dodson, and A. Dunaif. 1999. Prevalence and Predictors of Risk for Type 2 Diabetes Mellitus and Impaired Glucose Tolerance in Polycystic Ovary Syndrome: A Prospective, Controlled Study in 254 Affected Women. *The Journal of Clinical Endocrinology & Metabolism* 84(1): 165–169.

Leslie, Julia. 1996. Menstruation Myths. In *Myth and Mythmaking: Continuous Evolution in Indian Tradition*. Julia Leslie, ed. Pp. 87–105. London: Routledge.

Liboiron, Max. 2016. Redefining Pollution and Action: The Matter of Plastics. *Journal of Material Culture* 21(1): 87–110.

Liboiron, Max, Manuel Tironi, and Nerea Calvillo. 2018. Toxic Politics: Acting in a Permanently Polluted World. *Social Studies of Science* 48(3): 331–349.

Liddle, Joanna and Rama Joshi. 1986. *Daughters of Independence: Gender, Caste, and Class in India*. Rutgers: Rutgers University Press.

Lock, Margaret. 1993. *Encounters with Aging: Mythologies of Menopause in Japan and North America*. Berkeley: University of California Press.

Lock, Margaret and Patricia Kaufert. 2001. Menopause, Local Biologies, and Cultures of Aging. *American Journal of Human Biology* 13(4): 494–504.

Lock, Margaret and Vinh-Kim Nguyen. 2010. *An Anthropology of Biomedicine*. Oxford: Wiley–Blackwell.

Lora–Wainwright, Ann. 2010. An Anthropology of 'Cancer Villages': Villagers' Perspectives and the Politics of Responsibility. *Journal of Contemporary China* 19(63): 79–99.

143

Lora–Wainwright, Ann. 2013. The Inadequate Life: Rural Industrial Pollution and Lay Epidemiology in China. *The China Quarterly* 214: 302–320.

Luhar, Shammi, Poppy Alice Carson Mallinson, Lynda Clarke, and Sanjay Kinra. 2018. Trends in the Socioeconomic Patterning of Overweight/Obesity in India: A Repeated Cross-Sectional Study Using Nationally Representative Data. *British Medical Journal Open* 8(10): e023935.

Lukose, Ritty. 2009. *Liberalization's Children: Gender, Youth, and Consumer Citizenship in Globalizing India*. Durham: Duke University Press.

MacKendrick, Norah A. 2010. Media Framing of Body Burdens: Precautionary Consumption and the Individualization of Risk. *Sociological Inquiry* 80(1): 126–149.

Mahindra, Anand G. 2006. A Mature Society Embraces Prosperity. *Far Eastern Economic Review* 169(9): 44–46.

Majumdar, Soumita. 2010. PCOD Is Staring at More Number of Adolescent Girls. *Daily News & Analysis*, Aug 10. https://www.dnaindia.com/bangalore/report-pcod-is-staring-at-more-number-of-adolescent-girls-1427851, accessed Feb 24, 2021.

Mankekar, Purnima. 2004. Dangerous Desires: Television and Erotics in Late Twentieth-Century India. *The Journal of Asian Studies* 63(2): 403–431.

Mathur, H. B., H. C. Agarwal, Sapna Johnson, and Nirmaili Saikia. 2005. *Analysis of Pesticide Residues in Blood Samples from Villages of Punjab*. New Delhi: CSE.

Mazzarella, William. 2003. *Shoveling Smoke: Advertising and Globalization in Contemporary India*. New Delhi: Oxford University Press.

Mazzarella, William. 2005. Middle Class. In *South Asia Keywords*. Rachel Dwyer, ed. London: School of Oriental and African Studies. https://www.soas.ac.uk/ssai/keywords/file24808.pdf, accessed Oct 18, 2014.

McDermott, Robyn. 1998. Ethics, Epidemiology and the Thrifty Gene: Biological Determinism as a Health Hazard. *Social Science & Medicine* 47(9): 1189–1195.

McGuire, Meredith Lindsay. 2011. "How to Sit, How to Stand": Bodily Practice and the New Urban Middle Class. In *A Companion to the Anthropology of India*. Isabelle Clark-Decès, ed. Pp. 117–136. Malden: Wiley-Blackwell.

McKeigue, P. M., B. Shah, and M. G. Marmot. 1991. Relation of Central Obesity and Insulin Resistance with High Diabetes Prevalence and Cardiovascular Risk in South Asians. *The Lancet* 337(8738): 382–386.

Mehta, Bhamini and Shagufa Kapadia. 2008. Experiences of Childlessness in an Indian Context: A Gender Perspective. *Indian Journal of Gender Studies* 15(3): 437–460.

Mendenhall, Emily, Roopa Shivashankar, Nikhil Tandon, Mohammed K. Ali, K. M. Venkat Narayan, and Dorairaj Prabhakaran. 2012. Stress and Diabetes in Socioeconomic Context: A Qualitative Study of Urban Indians. *Social Science & Medicine* 75(12): 2522–2529.

Millard, Ann V. 1990. The Place of the Clock in Pediatric Advice: Rationales, Cultural Themes, and Impediments to Breastfeeding. *Social Science & Medicine* 31(2): 211–221.

Misra, Anoop, Debashish Chaudhary, Naval K. Vikram, Vivek Mittal, J. Rama Devi, Ravindra Pandey, Nidhi Khanna, Rekha Sharma, and Sharada Peshin. 2002. Insulin Resistance and Clustering of Atherogenic Risk Factors in Women Belonging to Low Socio-economic Strata in Urban Slums of North India. *Diabetes Research and Clinical Practice* 56(1): 73–75.

Misra, Anoop and Lokesh Khurana. 2008. Obesity and the Metabolic Syndrome in Developing Countries. *The Journal of Clinical Endocrinology & Metabolism* 93(11): S9–S30.

Misra, A., R. M. Pandey, J. Rama Devi, R. Sharma, N. K. Vikram, and Nidhi Khanna. 2001. High Prevalence of Diabetes, Obesity and Dyslipidaemia in Urban Slum Population in Northern India. *International Journal of Obesity* 25(11): 1722–1729.

Misra, A. et al. 2009. Consensus Statement for Diagnosis of Obesity, Abdominal Obesity and the Metabolic Syndrome for Asian Indians and Recommendations for Physical Activity, Medical and Surgical Management. *Journal of the Association of Physicians of India* 57: 163–170.

Mody, Perveez. 2002. Love and the Law: Love Marriage in Delhi. *Modern Asian Studies* 36(1): 223–256.

Mohan, Anjana Ranjit et al. 2017. Prevalence of Diabetes and Prediabetes in 15 states of India: Results from the ICMR–INDIAB Population-Based Cross-Sectional Study. *The Lancet: Diabetes & Endocrinology* 5(8): 585–596.

Mohan, Vathsala, Sandeep Sreedharan, R. Deepa, B. Shah, and C. Varghese. 2007. Epidemiology of Type 2 Diabetes: Indian Scenario. *Indian Journal of Medical Research* 125(3): 217–230.

Montoya, Michael. 2007. Bioethnic Conscription: Gene, Race, and Mexicana/o Ethnicity in Diabetes Research. *Cultural Anthropology* 22(1): 94–128.

Moran, Lisa, Grant Brinkworth, Manny Noakes, and Robert Norman. 2006. Effects of Lifestyle Modification in Polycystic Ovarian Syndrome. *Reproductive Biomedicine Online* 12(5): 569–578.

Mukerjee, Anjali. 2012. Weight Loss—Solution for PCOD. *Hindustan Times*, Dec 11. https://www.hindustantimes.com/health-and-fitness/weight-loss-a-solution-for-pcod/story-aCYSqAcELeKf6ytrKeIlZP.html, accessed Feb 24, 2021.

Mulgaonkar, V. B. 2001. *A Research and an Intervention Programme on Women's Reproductive Health in Slums of Mumbai.* Mumbai: Sujeevan Trust.

Munshi, Shoma. 2001. Marvellous Me: The Beauty Industry and the Construction of the "Modern" Indian Woman. In *Images of the "Modern Woman" in Asia. Global Media, Local Meanings.* Shoma Munshi, ed. Pp. 78–93. Richmond, Surrey: Curzon Press.

Murphy, Michelle. 2006. *Sick Building Syndrome and the Problem of Uncertainty: Environmental Politics, Technoscience, and Women Workers.* Durham: Duke University Press.

Murphy, Michelle. 2017. Alterlife and Decolonial Chemical Relations. *Cultural Anthropology* 32(4): 494–503.

Nading, Alex. 2020. Living in a Toxic World. *Annual Review of Anthropology* 49: 209–224.

Nagesh, B. S. 2012. The Food and Grocery Market. In *Businessworld Marketing Whitebook 2012–2013.* P. Datta, ed. Pp. 187–205. New Delhi: ABP.

Nash, Linda. 2006. *Inescapable Ecologies: A History of Disease, Environment, and Knowledge.* Berkeley: University of California Press.

Nashrulla, Tasneem. 2010. Don't Ignore Warning Signs. *Hindustan Times*, Jun 7. https://www.hindustantimes.com/mumbai/don-t-ignore-warning-signs/story-YRuzDqNXAAtOIEKRVnxidL.html, accessed Feb 24, 2021.

Navarro, Vicente (ed.). 2002. *The Political Economy of Social Inequalities: Consequences for Health and Quality of Life.* Amityville: Baywood Press.

Nichols, Carly. 2017. Millets, Milk and Maggi: Contested Processes of the Nutrition Transition in Rural India. *Agriculture and Human Values* 34: 871–885.

Nichter, Mark. 1980. The Layperson's Perception of Medicine as a Perspective into the Utilization of Multiple Therapy Systems in the Indian Context. *Social Science & Medicine* 14(4): 225–233.

Nichter, Mark. 1981. Idioms of Distress: Alternatives in the Expression of Psychosocial Distress: A Case Study from South India. *Culture, Medicine and Psychiatry* 5(4): 379–408.

Nichter, Mark. 1989. Pharmaceuticals, Health Commodification, and Social Relations: Ramifications for Primary Health Care. In *Anthropology and International Health. Asian Case Studies*. Mark Nichter, ed. Pp. 233–276. Dordrecht: Kluwer Academic Publishers.

Nichter, Mark. 1996. Pharmaceuticals, the Commodification of Health, and the Health Care-Medicine Use Transition. In *Anthropology and International Health. Asian Case Studies*. Mark Nichter and Mimi Nichter, eds. Pp. 268–333. New York: Routledge.

Nichter, Mark. 2001. The Political Ecology of Health in India: Indigestion as Sign and Symptom of Defective Modernization. In *Healing Powers and Modernity: Traditional Medicine, Shamanism, and Science in Asian Societies*. Linda H. Connor and Geoffrey Samuel, eds. Pp. 85–106. Westport and London: Bergin & Garvey.

Nichter, Mark. 2003. Harm Reduction: A Core Concern for Medical Anthropology. In *Risk, Culture, and Health Inequality*. Barbara Herr Harthorn and Laury Oaks, eds. Pp. 13–33. Westport: Praeger.

Nichter, Mark and David Van Sickle. 2002. The Challenges of India's Health and Health Care Transitions. In *India Briefing. Quickening the Pace of Change*. Alyssa Ayres and Philip Oldenburg, eds. Pp. 159–196. Armonk: M. E. Sharpe.

Nichter, Mark and Mimi Nichter. 1996. Modern Methods of Fertility Regulation: When and for Whom Are They Appropriate? In *Anthropology and International Health: Asian Case Studies*. Mark Nichter and Mimi Nichter, eds. Pp. 70–108. New York: Routledge.

Nisbett, Nicholas. 2007. Friendship, Consumption, Morality: Practising Identity, Negotiating Hierarchy in Middle-Class Bangalore. *Journal of the Royal Anthropological Institute* 13(4): 935–950.

Nixon, Rob. 2011. *Slow Violence and the Environmentalism of the Poor*. Cambridge: Harvard University Press.

Osella, Caroline. 2012. Desires Under Reform: Contemporary Reconfigurations of Family, Marriage, Love and Gendering in a Transnational South Indian Matrilineal Muslim Community. *Culture and Religion* 13(2): 241–264.

Osella, Caroline and Fillipo Osella. 2006. *Men and Masculinities in South India*. London: Anthem Press.

Padamsee, Tasleem Juana. 2011. The Pharmaceutical Corporation and the "Good Work" of Managing Women's Bodies. *Social Science and Medicine* 72(8): 1342–1350.

Paeratakul, S., J. C. Lovejoy, D. H. Ryan, and G. A. Bray. 2002. The Relation of Gender, Race and Socioeconomic Status to Obesity and Obesity Comorbidities in a Sample of US Adults. *International Journal of Obesity* 26: 1205–1210.

Pal, Somita. 2013. PCOS Hitting the Young. *Daily News & Analysis*, Mar 8. https://www.dnaindia.com/mumbai/report-pcos-hitting-the-young-1808737, accessed Feb 24, 2021.

Palioura, Eleni and Evanthia Diamanti-Kandarakis. 2015. Polycystic Ovary Syndrome (PCOS) and Endocrine Disrupting Chemicals (EDCs). *Reviews in Endocrine and Metabolic Disorders* 16: 365–371.

Patel, Sujata. 2004. Bombay/Mumbai: Globalization, Inequalities, and Politics. In *World Cities Beyond the West: Globalization, Development and Inequality.* Josef Gugler, ed. Pp. 328–347. Cambridge: Cambridge University Press.

Pathak, Gauri. 2014. "Presentable": The Body and Neoliberal Subjecthood in Contemporary India. *Social Identities: Journal for the Study of Race, Nation, and Culture* 20(4–5): 314–329.

Pathak, Gauri. 2020. Permeable Persons and Plastic Packaging in India: From Biomoral Substance Exchange to Chemotoxic Transmission. *Journal of the Royal Anthropological Institute* 26(4): 751–765.

Pearson, Natalie Obiko and Rakteem Katakey. 2014. India's Diesel Cars Are Proving Lethal. *Bloomberg Businessweek*, Mar 6.

Pepper, Daniel. 2007. Dead Rivers and Raw Sewage: Choking on Pollution in India. *Spiegel Online International*, Jul 6. http://www.spiegel.de/international/world/dead-rivers-and-raw-sewage-choking-on-pollution-in-india-a-493033.html, accessed Jul 8, 2014.

Pine, Jason. 2016. Last Chance Incorporated. *Cultural Anthropology* 31(2): 297–318.

Pingali, Prabhu. 2007. Westernization of Asian Diets and the Transformation of Food Systems: Implications for Research and Policy. *Food Policy* 32(3): 281–298.

Pinto, Sarah. 2011. Rational Love, Relational Medicine: Psychiatry and the Accumulation of Precarious Kinship. *Culture, Medicine, and Psychiatry* 35: 376–395.

Pomeroy, Emma, Veena Mushrif–Tripathy, Tim Cole, Jonathan C. K. Wells, and Jay T. Stock. 2019. Ancient Origins of Low Lean Mass among South Asians and Implications for Modern Type 2 Diabetes Susceptibility. *Scientific Reports* 9: 10515.

Popkin, Barry. 1993. Nutritional Patterns and Transitions. *Population and Development Review* 19(1): 138–157.

Popkin, Barry. 2001. The Nutrition Transition and Obesity in the Developing World. *The Journal of Nutrition* 131(3): 871S–873S.

Popkin, Barry. 2006. Global Nutrition Dynamics: The World Is Shifting Rapidly Toward a Diet Linked with Noncommunicable Diseases. *American Journal of Clinical Nutrition* 84(2): 289–298.

Prabhakaran, Dorairaj, Salim Yusuf, Shamir Mehta, Janice Pogue, Alvaro Avezum, Andrzej Budaj, Leszek Cerumzynski, Marcus Flather, Keith Fox, David Hunt, Liu Lisheng, Matyas Keltai, Alexander Parkhomenko, Prem Pais, Srinath Reddy, Mikhail Ruda, Tan Hiquing, and Zhu Jun. 2005. Two-Year Outcomes in Patients Admitted with Non-ST Elevation Acute Coronary Syndrome: Results of the OASIS Registry 1 and 2. *Indian Heart Journal* 57(3): 217–225.

Prakash, Gyan. 1999. *Another Reason: Science and the Imagination of Modern India.* Princeton: Princeton University Press.

Quesada, James, Laurie Kain Hart, and Philippe Bourgois. 2011. Structural Vulnerability and Health: Latino Migrant Laborers in the United States. *Medical Anthropology* 30(4): 339–362.

Radhakrishnan, Smitha. 2009. Professional Women, Good Families: Respectable Femininity and the Cultural Politics of a "New" India. *Qualitative Sociology* 32: 195–212.

Radhakrishnan, Smitha. 2011. *Appropriately Indian: Gender and Culture in a New Transnational Class*. Durham and London: Duke University Press.

Raheja, Gloria Goodwin and Ann Grodzins Gold. 1994. *Listen to the Heron's Words: Reimagining Gender and Kinship in North India*. Berkeley: University of California Press.

Rajagopal, Arvind. 2001. Thinking About the New Indian Middle Class. Gender, Advertising and Politics in an Age of Globalisation. In *Signposts: Gender Issues in Post-Independence India*. Rajeswari Sunder Rajan, ed. Pp. 57–99. New Brunswick: Rutgers University Press.

Ramachandran, A. 2005. Epidemiology of Diabetes in India—Three Decades of Research. *Journal of the Association of Physicians of India* 53: 34–38.

Rao, Vyjayanthi. 2006. Risk and the City: Bombay, Mumbai and Other Theoretical Departures. *India Review* 5(2): 220–232.

Ravichandran, Nalini. 2014. When Hormones Go Awry. *India Today*, Jul 15. https://www.indiatoday.in/lifestyle/health/story/hormones-go-awry-hormonal-disorder-pcos-polycystic-ovarian-syndrome-200429-2014-07-15, accessed Feb 24, 2021.

Razak, Fahad, Sonia S. Anand, Vladimir Vuksan, B. Davis, R. Jacobs, Koon K. Teo, and Salim Yusuf. 2005. Ethnic Differences in the Relationships Between Obesity and Glucose-Metabolic Abnormalities: A Cross-Sectional Population-Based Study. *International Journal of Obesity* 29: 656–667.

Reddy, Srinath K., B. Shah, C. Varghese, and A. Ramadoss. 2005. Responding to the Threat of Chronic Diseases in India. *The Lancet* 366(9498): 1744–1749.

Reddy, Sunita and Imrana Qadeer. 2010. Medical Tourism in India: Progress or Predicament? *Economic & Political Weekly* 45(20): 69–75.

Reddy, Sunita, Tulsi Patel, Malene Tanderup Kristensen, and Birgitte Bruun Nielsen. 2018. Surrogacy in India: Political and Commercial Framings. In *Cross-Cultural Comparisons on Surrogacy and Egg Donation. Interdisciplinary Perspectives from India, Germany, and Israel*. Sayani Mitra, Silke Schicktanz, and Tulsi Patel, eds. Pp. 153–179. Cham: Palgrave Macmillan.

Riessman, Catherine Kohler. 2000. Stigma and Everyday Resistance Practices: Childless Woman in South India. *Gender & Society* 14(1): 111–135.

Roberts, Elizabeth F. S. 2015. Bio-Ethnography: A Collaborative, Methodological Experiment in Mexico City. *Somatosphere*, Feb 26. http://somatosphere.net/2015/bio-ethnography.html/, accessed Jul 16, 2021.

Roberts, Elizabeth F. S. 2017. What Gets Inside: Violent Entanglements and Toxic Boundaries in Mexico City. *Cultural Anthropology* 32(4): 592–619.

Rodrik, Dani and Arvind Subramaniam. 2004. From "Hindu Growth" to Productivity Surge: The Mystery of the Indian Growth Transition. *Faculty Research Working Papers Series*. John F. Kennedy School of Government, Harvard University.

Rokade, S. and A. Mane. 2009. A Study of Age at Menarche, the Secular Trend and Factors Associated with It. *Internet Journal of Biological Anthropology* 3(2). https://ispub.com/IJBA/3/2/7469, accessed Feb 8, 2021.

Rose, Nikolas. 2006. *The Politics of Life Itself: Biomedicine, Power, and Subjectivity in the Twenty-First Century*. Princeton: Princeton University Press.

Rotterdam ESHRE/ASRM-Sponsored PCOS Consensus Workshop Group. 2004. Revised 2003 Consensus on Diagnostic Criteria and Long-Term Health Risks Related to Polycystic Ovary Syndrome (PCOS). *Human Reproduction* 19(1): 41–47.

Runkle, Susan. 2003. Bollywood, Beauty, and the Corporate Construction of "International Standards" in Post-Liberalization Bombay. *Sagar: South Asian Graduate Research Journal* 11: 37–57.

Rutkowska, Aleksandra and Dominik Rachoń. 2014. Bisphenol A (BPA) and Its Potential Role in the Pathogenesis of the Polycystic Ovary Syndrome (PCOS). *Gynecological Endocrinology* 30(4): 260–265.

S., Anandhi. 1998. Reproductive Bodies and Regulated Sexuality. Birth Control Debates in Early 20th Century Tamilnadu. In *A Question of Silence: The Sexual Economics of Modern India*. Mary John and Janaki Nair, eds. Pp. 139–166. New Delhi: Kali for Women.

Salans, Lester B., Samuel W. Cushman, and Rodger E. Weismann. 1973. Studies of Human Adipose Tissue. Adipose Cell Size and Number in Nonobese and Obese Patients. *The Journal of Clinical Investigation* 52(4): 929–941.

Samulowitz, Anke, Ida Gremyr, Erik Eriksson, and Gunnel Hensing. 2018. "Brave Men" and "Emotional Women": A Theory-Guided Literature Review on Gender Bias in Health Care and Gendered Norms towards Patients with Chronic Pain. *Pain Research and Management*. https://www.hindawi.com/journals/prm/2018/6358624/

Sancho, David. 2016. *Youth, Class and Education in Urban India. The Year That Can Break or Make You*. London: Routledge.

Sandelowski, Margarete. 1991. Compelled to Try: The Never-Enough Quality of Conceptive Technology. *Medical Anthropology Quarterly* 5(1): 29–47.

Sankararamakrishnan, N., A. Kumar Sharma, and R. Sanghi. 2005. Organochlorine and Organophosphorous Pesticide Residues in Ground Water and Surface Waters of Kanpur, Uttar Pradesh, India. *Environment International* 31(1): 113–120.

Saper, Robert B., Russell S. Phillips, Anusha Sehgal, Nadia Khouri, Roger B. Davis, Janet Paquin, Venkatesh Thuppil, and Stefanos N. Kales. 2008. Lead, Mercury, and Arsenic in US- and Indian-Manufactured Ayurvedic Medicines Sold via the Internet. *Journal of the American Medical Association* 300(8): 915–923.

Schmidt, Christian, Tobias Krauth, and Stephan Wagner. 2017. Export of Plastic Debris by Rivers into the Sea. *Environmental Science and Technology* 51(21): 12246–12253.

Seymour, Susan. 1999. *Women, Family, and Child-Care in India: A World in Transition*. Cambridge: Cambridge University Press.

Shapiro, Nicholas. 2015. Attuning to the Chemosphere: Domestic Formaldehyde, Bodily Reasoning, and the Chemical Sublime. *Cultural Anthropology* 30(3): 368–393.

Sharangpani, Mukta. 2010. Browsing for Bridegrooms: Matchmaking and Modernity in Mumbai. *Indian Journal of Gender Studies* 17(2): 249–276.

Sharma, Shalendra. 2003. India's Economic Liberalization: A Progress Report. *Current History* 102(663): 176–179.

Sheehan, Michael T. 2004. Polycystic Ovarian Syndrome: Diagnosis and Management. *Clinical Medicine and Research* 2(1): 13–27.

Shetty, Prakash. 2002. Nutrition Transition in India. *Public Health Nutrition* 5(1A): 175–182.

Simonelli, J. M. 1987. Defective Modernization and Health in Mexico. *Social Science & Medicine* 24(1): 23–36.

Singare, Pravin U. 2016. Carcinogenic and Endocrine-Disrupting PAHs in the Aquatic Ecosystem of India. *Environmental Monitoring and Assessment* 188: 599.

Singer, Linda. 1989. Bodies-Pleasures-Powers. *Differences* 1(1): 45–65.

Singer, Merill and Scott Clair. 2003. Syndemics and Public Health: Reconceptualizing Disease in Bio-Social Context. *Medical Anthropology Quarterly* 17(4): 423–441.

Singh, Holly Donahue. 2020. Numbering Others: Religious Demography, Identity, and Fertility Management Experiences in Contemporary India. *Social Science & Medicine* 254: 112534.

Singh, Alka, L. K. Dhaliwal, and Amandeep Kaur. 1997. Infertility in a Primary Health Centre of Northern India: A Follow Up Study. *Journal of Family Welfare* 42(1): 51–56.

Singh, Kavita, K. M. Venkat Narayan, and Karen Eggleston. 2019. Economic Impact of Diabetes in South Asia: The Magnitude of the Problem. *Current Diabetes Reports* 19(34). https://doi.org/10.1007/s11892-019-1146-1

Singh, Upma, Shikha Singh, Rishikesh K. Tiwari, and Ravi S. Pandey. 2018. Pollution Due to Discharge of Industrial Effluents with Special Reference to Uttar Pradesh, India—A Review. *International Archive of Applied Sciences and Technology* 9(4): 111–121.

Skrbis, Zlatko, Gavin Kendall, and Ian Woodward. 2004. Locating Cosmopolitanism Between Humanist Ideal and Grounded Social Category. *Theory, Culture & Society* 21(6): 115–136.

Solomon, Harris. 2016. The Thin–Fat Indian. In *Metabolic Living: Food, Fat, and the Absorption of Illness in India*. Pp. 31–64. Durham: Duke University Press.

Sosale, Bhavana, Aravind R. Sosale, Anjana R. Mohan, Prasanna M. Kumar, Banshi Saboo, and Sai Kandula. 2016. Cardiovascular Risk Factors, Micro and Macrovascular Complications at Diagnosis in Patients with Young Onset Type 2 Diabetes in India: CINDI 2. *Indian Journal of Endocrinology and Metabolism* 20(1): 114–118.

Soulez, Benoit, Dewailly Didier, and Robert L. Rosenfield. 1996. Polycystic Ovary Syndrome: A Multidisciplinary Challenge. *Endocrinologist* 6(1):19–29.

Spiegel, Karine, Esra Tasali, Rachel Leproult, and Eve Van Cauter. 2009. Effects of Poor and Short Sleep on Glucose Metabolism and Obesity Risk. *Nature Reviews Endocrinology* 5: 253–261.

Srinivas, Mysore Narasimhachar. 1994. Sociology in India and Its Future. *Sociological Bulletin* 43(1): 9–19.

Srivastava, Ashutosh K., Purushottam Trivedi, M. K. Srivastava, M. Lohani, and Laxman Prasad Srivastava. 2011. Monitoring of Pesticide Residues in Market Basket Samplers of Vegetable from Lucknow City, India: QuEChERS Method. *Environmental Monitoring and Assessment* 176: 465–472.

Srivastava, Sanjay. 2007. *Passionate Modernity: Sexuality, Class and Consumption in India*. New Delhi: Routledge Publishers.

Starka, L., M. Duskova, I. Cermakova, J. Vrbikova, and M. Hill. 2005. Premature Androgenic Alopecia and Insulin Resistance. Male Equivalent of Polycystic Ovary Syndrome? *Endocrine Regulations* 39(4): 127–131.

Stokken, Roar. 2009. The Patient Educated Patient: A Health-Care Asset of Problem? *Social Theory & Health* 7: 81–99.

Suryanarayan, Deepa. 2007. Lifestyle Disease Deals Fair Sex an Unfair Blow. *Daily News & Analysis*, Apr 13. https://www.dnaindia.com/mumbai/report-lifestyle-disease-deals-fair-sex-an-unfair-blow-1090567, accessed Feb 24, 2021.

Swaminathan, Sumathi, Sumithra Selvam, Tinku Thomas, Anura Kurpad, and Mario Vaz. 2011. Longitudinal Trends in Physical Activity Patterns in Selected Urban South Indian School Children. *Indian Journal of Medical Research* 134(2): 174–180.

Talukdar, Jaita. 2012. Thin But Not Skinny: Women Negotiating the "Never Too Thin" Body Ideal in Urban India. *Women's Studies International Forum* 35(2): 109–118.

Thapan, Meenakshi. 2004. Embodiment and Identity in Contemporary Society: Femina and the "New" Indian Woman. *Contributions to Indian Sociology* 38(3): 411–444.

Tillin, Therese, Naveed Sattar, Ian F. Godsland, Alun Hughes, Nishi Chaturvedi, and Nita Gandhi Farouhi. 2015. Ethnicity-Specific Obesity Cut-Points in the Development of Type 2 Diabetes – A Prospective Study Including Three Ethnic Groups in the United Kingdom. *Diabetic Medicine* 32(2): 226–234.

Times of India. 2012. Modern Lifestyle Increases PCOS Cases. *Times of India*, Jan 20. https://timesofindia.indiatimes.com/city/nagpur/Modern-lifestyle-increases-PCOS-cases/articleshow/11561204.cms, accessed Feb 24, 2021.

Tironi, Manuel. 2018. Hypo-Interventions: Intimate Activism in Toxic Environments. *Social Studies of Science* 48(3): 438–455.

Tiwari, M., S. K. Sahu, and G. G. Pandit. 2016. Distribution and Estrogenic Potential of Endocrine Disrupting Chemicals (EDCs) in Estuarine Sediments from Mumbai, India. *Environmental Science and Pollution Research* 23: 18789–18799.

Uberoi, Patricia. 2001. Imagining the Family: An Ethnography of Viewing Hum Aapke Hain Koun...! In *Pleasure and the Nation: The History, Politics and Consumption of Popular Culture in India*. Rachel Dwyer and Christopher Pinney, eds. Pp. 309–351. SOAS Studies on South Asia. New Delhi: Oxford University Press.

Uberoi, Patricia. 2008. Aspirational Weddings: The Bridal Magazine and the Canons of "Decent Marriage". In *Patterns of Middle Class Consumption in India and China*. Christopher Jaffrelot and Peter van der Veer, eds. Pp. 230–262. New Delhi: Sage Publications.

Unisa, Sayeed. 1999. Childlessness in Andhra Pradesh, India: Treatment Seeking and Consequences. *Reproductive Health Matters* 7(13): 54–64.

United Nations Development Programme. 2011. India Factsheet: Economic and Human Development Indicators. www.in.undp.org/content/dam/india/docs/india_factsheet_economic_n_hdi.pdf, accessed Nov 9, 2014.

Unnithan, Maya. 2010. Infertility and Assisted Reproductive Technologies (ARTs) in a Globalising India: Ethics, Medicalisation, and Agency. *Asian Bioethics Review* 2(1): 3–18.

Unnithan, Maya. 2019. *Fertility, Health, and Reproductive Politics: Re-imagining Rights in India*. London: Routledge.

Upadhyay, R. P. 2012. An Overview of the Burden of Noncommunicable Diseases in India. *Iran Journal of Public Health* 41: 1–8.

Vandenberg, Laura N. 2014. Low-Dose Effects of Hormones and Endocrine Disruptors. In *Endocrine Disrupters*. G. Litwack, ed. Pp. 129–165. San Diego: Elsevier.

Vedwan, Neeraj. 2007. Pesticides in Coca-Cola and Pepsi: Consumerism, Brand Image, and Public Interest in a Globalizing India. *Cultural Anthropology* 22(4): 659–684.

van der Veer, Peter. 2001. *Imperial Encounters: Religion and Modernity in India and Britain*. Princeton: Princeton University Press.

Venkatesh, Alladi. 1994. India's Changing Consumer Economy: A Cultural Perspective. In *NA – Advances in Consumer Research*. Chris T. Allen and Deborah R. John, eds. Pp. 323–328. Provo, UT: Association for Consumer Research.

Verma, Suman, Deepali Sharma, and Reed Larson. 2002. School Stress in India: Effects on Time and Daily Emotions. *International Journal of Behavioral Development* 26(6): 500–508.

Vogel, Sarah. 2012. *Is It Safe?: BPA and the Struggle to Define the Safety of Chemicals.* Berkeley: University of California Press.

Wadley, Susan. 2002. One Straw from a Broom Cannot Sweep: The Ideology and Practice of the Joint Family in Rural North India. In *Everyday Life in South Asia.* Diane P. Mines and Sarah Lamb, eds. Pp. 11–22. Bloomington: Indiana University Press.

Washbrook, David. 1997. From Comparative Sociology to Global History: Britain and India in the Pre-History of Modernity. *Journal of the Economic and Social History of the Orient* 40(4): 410–443.

Wasir, Jasjeet Singh and Anoop Misra. 2004. The Metabolic Syndrome in Asian Indians: Impact of Nutritional and Socio-Economic Transition in India. *Metabolic Syndrome and Related Disorders* 2(1): 14–23.

Weaver, Lesley Jo and Emily Mendenhall. 2014. Applying Syndemics and Chronicity: Interpretations from Studies of Poverty, Depression, and Diabetes. *Medical Anthropology* 33(2): 92–108.

Wells, Jonathan C. K., Emma Pomeroy, Subhash R. Walimbe, Barry M. Popkin, and Chittaranjan S. Yajnik. 2016. The Elevated Susceptibility to Diabetes in India: An Evolutionary Perspective. *Frontiers in Public Health* 4: 145.

van Wessel, Margit. 2004. Talking About Consumption. How an Indian Middle Class Dissociates from Middle Class Life. *Cultural Dynamics* 16(1): 93–116.

Wijeyaratne, C., S. A. Dilini Udayangani, and A. Balen. 2013. Ethnic-specific Polycystic Ovary Syndrome: Epidemiology, Significance, and Implications. *Expert Review of Endocrinology and Metabolism* 8(1): 71–79.

Wild, Sarah, Gojka Roglic, Anders Green, Richard Sicree, and Hilary King. 2004. Global Prevalence of Diabetes: Estimates for the Year 2000 and Projections for 2030. *Diabetes Care* 27(5): 1047–1053.

Wilhite, Harold. 2008. *Consumption and the Transformation of Everyday Life.* London: Palgrave Macmillan.

Wilson, Caroline. 2010. "Eating, Eating Is Always There": Food, Consumerism and Cardiovascular Disease. Some Evidence from Kerala, South India. *Anthropology & Medicine* 17(3): 261–275.

World Bank. 2018. GDP, PPP (Current International $)—India. *World Bank Development Indicators Database.* https://data.worldbank.org/indicator/NY.GDP.MKTP.PP.CD?locations=IN, accessed Jun 5, 2020.

World Bank Group and Institute for Health Metrics and Evaluation. 2016. *The Cost of Air Pollution. Strengthening the Economic Case for Action.* Washington: World Bank Group and Institute for Health Metrics and Evaluation. http://documents.worldbank.org/curated/en/781521473177013155/pdf/108141-REVISED-Cost-of-PollutionWebCORRECTEDfile.pdf, accessed Jun 5, 2020.

Wylie, Sara. 2018. *Fractivism: Corporate Bodies and Chemical Bonds.* Durham, NC: Duke University Press.

Xavier, Denis, Prem Pais, P. J. Deveraux, Changchun Xie, Dorairaj Prabhakaran, K. Srinath Reddy, Rajeev Gupta, Prashant Joshi, Prafulla Kerkar, S. Thanikachalam, K. K. Haridas, T. M. Jaison, Sudhir Naik, A. K. Maity, and Salim Yusuf. 2008. Treatment and Outcomes of Acute Coronary Syndromes in India (CREATE): A Prospective Analysis of Registry Data. *The Lancet* 371(9622): 1435–1442.

Xu, Zhiye, Dan Yu, Xueyao Yin, Fenping Zheng, and Hong Li. 2017. Socioeconomic Status Is Associated with Global Diabetes Prevalence. *Oncotarget* 8(27): 44434–44439.

Yadav, Ishwar Chandra, Ningombam Linthoingambi Devi, Jabir Hussain Syed, Zhineng Cheng, Jun Li, Gan Zhang, and Kevin C. Jones. 2015. Current Status of Persistent Organic Pesticides Residues in Air, Water, and Soil, and Their Possible Effect on Neighboring Countries: A Comprehensive Review of India. *Science of the Total Environment* 511: 123–137.

Yajnik, Chittaranjan S. and John S. Yudkin. 2004. The Y–Y Paradox. *The Lancet* 363(9403): 163.

Yan, Yunxiang. 2010. The Chinese Path to Individualization. *The British Journal of Sociology* 61(3): 489–512.

Zimmermann, Francis. 1980. Rtu-Satmya: The Seasonal Cycle and the Principle of Appropriateness. *Social Science & Medicine* 14(2): 99–106.

INDEX

Pages in *italics* refer figures; pages in **bold** refer tables and pages followed by n refer notes.

154

For Product Safety Concerns and Information please contact our EU
representative GPSR@taylorandfrancis.com
Taylor & Francis Verlag GmbH, Kaufingerstraße 24, 80331 München, Germany